The Medical Student's Survival Guide 2

The Medical Student's Survival Guide 2
GOING CLINICAL

ELIZABETH COTTRELL
Foundation Year 1 Doctor
University Hospital of North Staffordshire

Radcliffe Publishing
Oxford • New York

Radcliffe Publishing Ltd
18 Marcham Road
Abingdon
Oxon OX14 1AA
United Kingdom

www.radcliffe-oxford.com
Electronic catalogue and worldwide online ordering facility.

British Library Cataloguing in Publication Data
A catalogue record for this book is available from the British Library.

ISBN-13 978 1 84619 213 5

Typeset by Egan Reid, Auckland, New Zealand
Printed and bound by TJI Digital, Padstow, Cornwall, UK

Contents

About the author

Elizabeth Cottrell, a Foundation Year 1 doctor, achieved MBChB (honours) while at medical school. She learnt a lot from co-writing her first book, *The Medical Student Career Handbook*, during her final year at medical school. This invaluable experience helped her to develop the *Medical Student Survival Guides* with national medical student involvement from the start. Elizabeth has drawn from her experiences, and those of other medical students, to provide useful information.

About the contributors

A few individuals deserve a special thank you for the vast amount of time, effort, work and support they have provided during the development of *The Medical Student's Survival Guides*. Each individual provided his or her time and expertise for nothing. The following individuals have been significantly involved in contributing to and critiquing chapters:

Dr Robert ('Bob') Clarke, Associate Dean for London Postgraduate Medical Education and 'a legend' to many medical students nationally. Also, thank you so much for your fantastic revision courses that helped me to become a doctor

Ms Kate Fraser, The University of Manchester Medical School

Dr Basma Hassan, Foundation Year 2 in the West Midlands Deanery

Ms Pauline Law, University of Dundee Medical School

Mr David Little, The University of Manchester Medical School

Mr Vishnu Madhok, University of Dundee Medical School

Dr Christele Rebora, Foundation Year 1 in the London Deanery

Mr Imran Sajid, The University of Manchester Medical School

Ms Laura Stevens, University of Dundee Medical School

Mr Paul White, University of St Andrews Medical School.

The following individuals contributed to the content of the *Survival Guide*: Allie Blair (The University of Liverpool), Rachel Boyce (University of Aberdeen), Nat Bradbrook (The University of Manchester), Zoe Cowan (The University of Leicester), Stephen Domek (University of East Anglia), David Douglas (University of Dundee), Esther Downham (University of Dundee), Kate Geraghty (The University of Leicester), Anna Kieslich (University of Dundee), Elizabeth Li (The University of Manchester), Jemima Miller (University College London), Oliver Shapter (University of Aberdeen), Ross Stewart (University of Dundee), Katie Thorne (The Hull York Medical School) and Alexandra Williams (University of Leeds).

Acknowledgements

Thank you to Dr Charlene Kennedy, Foundation Year 1, who encouraged me right at the start, when the *Survival Guide* was just a bubble of inspiration floating around my brain!

A thank you must also go to all my peers, colleagues and patients, who have provided me with the material, inspiration and experiences from which the book is written.

Lastly, a 'thank you' must go to my husband, my friend and my rock, Paul. Without his support, help and encouragement I would not be the happy wife, doctor, daughter and sister I am now.

CHAPTER 1

Introduction

Medicine is a vocation in which a doctor's knowledge, clinical skills and judgement are put in the service of protecting and restoring human well-being. This purpose is realised through a partnership between patient and doctor, one based on mutual respect, individual responsibility, and appropriate accountability.

In their day-to-day practice, doctors are committed to:

- integrity
- compassion
- altruism
- continuous improvement
- excellence
- working in partnership with members of the wider healthcare team.

These values, which underpin the science and practice of medicine, form the basis for a moral contract between the medical profession and society. Each party has a duty to work to strengthen the system of healthcare on which our collective human dignity depends.[1]

Medical school is fantastic, fun and fulfilling, but it is also tough. It may mean leaving home, fending for yourself for the first time, and it is mentally and physically challenging. The sister book to this, *The Medical Student's Survival Guide 1: the early years*, contains information on:

- medical school: the early days
- the people you will meet
- competitiveness, attitude and behaviour
- course structure
- learning and exams
- projects
- presentations
- money
- life away from medicine
- medical student socials

➨ when things go wrong in the early years
➨ how to get the most from the early years.

Similar to *The Medical Student's Survival Guide 1: the early years*, this book contains information on avoiding or managing the hazards of being a medical student, as identified by the medical student welfare surveys performed by the welfare subcommittee of the British Medical Association Medical Students' Committee (BMA MSC).

To succeed at medical school, you will work harder than you ever imagined. Your role and your presence will not always be appreciated, and you will have to mature quicker than many of your non-medical student peers. That said, medical school offers unique, intriguing and humbling experiences and opportunities. Few other degrees offer such insight into the lives of other people; this will make you very worldly wise. Medicine provides the buzz of success, the heartbreak of tragedies and mental and ethical challenges that go hand in hand with caring for, diagnosing, treating and managing patients and their friends and relatives.

The two *Medical Student's Survival Guides* have been developed to provide you with realistic insights into undergraduate training. *The Medical Student Survival Guide 1: the early years* contains information on the 'pre-clinical' years at university. The present *Survival Guide* is targeted at medical students entering the later years of their course, the majority of which will be delivered in a clinical setting. Although it is recognised that this split is not as clearly defined as implied in many medical schools, as some of you will receive clinical training from the first year, information contained in each *Survival Guide* will be signposted in both books to assist you to access the relevant information. The content has been informed by the enthusiasm, experiences, challenges and successes of the author and UK medical students. The *Survival Guides* may not always provide solutions but confirmation that your views, experiences and problems are not unique. Medicine and medical training is constantly changing and evolving. Therefore be proactive in finding the most up-to-date information that is available. The *Survival Guides* will signpost you to sources of current information on many of the topics covered.

The *Survival Guides* will not guarantee you a pass in your exams; however, they will provide you with information that will make the day-to-day experience of being a medical student much easier.

The *Survival Guides* contain quotes, thought bubbles, speech bubbles, arrows and stars:

➨ Quotes by UK medical students and literature: opinions, thoughts and advice that demonstrate the diversity of experiences that occur throughout medical training.
➨ Thought bubbles: examples of questions you should be asking yourself.
➨ Speech bubbles: questions commonly asked by tutors and examiners or useful phrases for you to try in the appropriate situations.

➡ Arrows: action you could take to further your experience, knowledge or practice.

➡ Stars: important and key knowledge that undergraduate students should grasp during medical school. Although not exhaustive, they will signpost important concepts and illustrate the level of understanding required of you.

The Appendix contains *Resources*, a directory containing comprehensive contact details for relevant organisations. Contact the organisations themselves for the most up-to-date, detailed and accurate information.

When applying to medical school many potential students declare a 'commitment to life-long learning' to demonstrate their desire to obtain a ticket to the marvellous journey that medicine provides. But what are the different routes, diversions and delays that today's medical students face, and are these causes for concern?

Medical students have to build a commendable CV in an environment where competitiveness and ambition is rife; passing written and clinical finals is simply not enough to join the bottom of the medical career ladder. So what can medical students do to distinguish themselves from a plethora of cloned colleagues? Get work published? Intercalate? Join their Medical School Committee? Evidently, competitiveness is an aspect of any career pathway, although there must surely be a feeling of déjà vu with personal statement writing and UCAS applications in the not-so-distant past for final-year students.

Another concern inherent among students is that of finances. Medical students are unusual as it is normal to spend up to six years completing an undergraduate degree. Demanding clinical timetables and gruelling revision regimens leave little scope for medical students to take on part-time employment. With several banks now offering professional loans of up to £20,000 and interest-free overdrafts, the opportunity for medical students to accumulate dangerously high levels of debt often receives attention from the media.

We must remember that the vocation of medicine is not a one-way ticket, and there are indeed many routes that may be taken before reaching the desired destination. Many doctors will reminisce about their turbulent journey and several places that they otherwise would never have had the opportunity to see while stopping en route. Although what remains evident is that 'commitment' must be a prerequisite before boarding. (*Vishnu Madhock, fourth-year medical student, Dundee*)

FURTHER READING

MacDonald R. Rhona's rules (on what being a medical student and doctor is all about). *StudentBMJ*. 2004; **12**: 458–9.

CHAPTER 2

Clinical years

> If you can stay calm, while all around you is in chaos, you probably haven't completely understood the seriousness of the situation.[1]

CLINICAL PLACEMENTS

> I spent the first two years concentrating on the theory of medicine, the study of the function and functioning of our wonderful bodies. Armed with oodles of meaningless knowledge we then hit the wards to see disease, illness and suffering.[2]

Clinical placements are the period of learning which occur in a clinical setting: a hospital, GP practice, local health centre or anywhere else healthcare and medicine are practised. Clinical placements may feature during any year of your course.

Your base hospital is the main hospital(s) that is (are) linked to your university. The majority of your clinical placements take place at your base hospital(s), although you may also study at district general hospitals and cottage hospitals.

Your medical school should provide you with details of your clinical placements at least one month in advance. This is particularly true for placements away from your base hospital, for which travel, accommodation and care of dependants may need to be arranged.[3] If you have dependants, or other special circumstances, you can request placements near to your base hospital.

Accommodation

Clinical placements at your base hospital usually do not present accommodation difficulties as the hospitals are close to the university. However, although medical schools offer many placements within commuting distance from the base hospital, sometimes this cannot be the case. Under these latter circumstances free accommodation should be available to you. The British Medical Association (BMA) states that medical students should have free accommodation in placements over three-quarters of an hour away, by public transport, from their base hospital.[3] The accommodation should meet with the Housing (Management of Houses in Multiple Occupations) Regulations (HIMOR) standards.[4]

Starting a new clinical placement

Before starting a new placement, make sure you know where the hospital is and how you will get there. Perhaps do a trial run at rush hour. Always arrange a meeting with your new tutor and use this to find out where your new ward or clinic is and who the staff members are. Use your pre-placement meeting to discuss the timetable, your objectives and any pre-placement work that is required.

Ask the staff where you should keep your belongings. Secure storage facilities should be available for all medical students. However, these are sometimes not available, accessible nor practicable, and thus of no use. Restrict what you take to a minimum and do not take any valuables. Leave credit cards and large amounts of cash at home; take just enough to buy lunch if necessary. If you are having major problems with secure storage of your belongings seek advice from your medical school. You have a right to be able to leave your belongings safely while you learn.

> Year 3 began with a four-week basic skills course, which involved attending lectures and demonstrations of useful techniques for use on the ward. The basic skills we were taught included taking a blood glucose measurement, general observations, examination of systems, basic life support, intramuscular and subcutaneous injections, and sessions on communication skills. Every student then had a 'ward week' at the different hospitals in the area. For this I was assisting nurses in a surgical ward. Daily duties involved helping to wash patients, changing bedding, recording observations and helping with the medicine trolley. Ward week provided an opportunity to see hospital life from a different angle; it really makes you appreciate how different members of staff (cleaners, occupational therapists, nurses) all contribute to the care of patients as well as doctors.
>
> Following the basic skills course all the students in my university started the 'Nutrition, Metabolism and Excretion' module. We were attached to two firms during the module, giving us seven weeks with each. We also spent a day in the community every week at a GP practice.
>
> In Year 3 we had students joining us from another university and we had students who had previously intercalated rejoining the main curriculum. As there were seven to eight students in my problem-based learning (PBL) group, and there were two sessions of PBL a week with an assigned tutor overseeing proceedings, it gave us the chance to get to know some new people. In my PBL group we all became really good

friends, having a laugh and a joke regularly, as well as competing at table football or going for group meals.

For the rest of the week (not spent in PBL) we attended clinical teaching sessions with the firm that my PBL group was attached to. Clinical teaching involved practising taking and presenting histories, performing examinations and some classroom-based teaching. It was very different to our teaching in years 1 and 2.

For the next module we are allocated to a new PBL group, with different students and a new tutor. *(Imran Sajid, fourth-year medical student, Manchester)*

Consideration for all

Always introduce yourself to new people on the ward; both staff and patients. Do not assume that everyone will recognise you are a medical student because you are wearing a white coat or because you have a stethoscope around your neck. Look around: pharmacists, specialist nurses and physiotherapists often wear at least one of these items.

A lot of your activities while on clinical placement are primarily for your benefit. Therefore do not make a nuisance of yourself. Those around you are either trying to work or get better; they do not want you messing around or being inconsiderate.

Most staff members appreciate enthusiastic students; however, they will never appreciate you asking lots of questions when they are very busy or doing drug rounds. Ask important questions which cannot wait and then note others down to ask during a quieter time.

If 'hundreds' of medical students attend their consultation it can be quite daunting for patients. Therefore, if your firm contains more than two medical students, arrange your individual timetables around one another to stop all of you turning up to clinic or ward rounds at the same time.

Hand-washing

Hand-washing should be mentioned on every page in this *Survival Guide* as it is a terrifically important weapon against the spread of infection. Your patients will not thank you if you forget to wash your hands and give them the infection that killed the patient in the next bed.

Wash your hands before and after EVERY patient contact – even just a handshake. In a hospital, GP surgery or clinic there is often a sink in every room. If not, an alcohol hand rub is now readily available and easy to use. Do not just wave your hands under some water or dab a little alcohol rub on for effect, really wash your hands thoroughly. If your hands are visibly dirty or contaminated, wash them with soap and water, rubbing them together for 15–20 seconds. If your hands are visibly clean, use an alcohol rub and rub your hands together until they are dry. When washing your hands pay particular attention to your thumbs, nails, wrists and in between your fingers as these are the areas most commonly missed.

Bleeps

The BMA states that bleeps should be available to all senior medical students. In reality, bleeps are only sometimes available (and rarely readily available) to medical students. You can always leave a telephone number if you want to be contacted to experience a certain event.

Computers

Computers are increasingly used in hospitals. Hospitals are moving towards paper-less systems, and referrals, reports, discharge documents, prescriptions and notes are being produced and displayed using computers. Keep abreast of changes to computer systems during your placements; regular training sessions are available and you should ask your medical school or tutor for more information on attending these if required.

All computer programs containing clinical information require passwords, and you must have and use your own. Your medical school will be able to tell you how to obtain any passwords you require (and are entitled to) when you are on your clinical placements. Never give your password to anyone else. Activities carried out under password are recorded and can be tracked. If someone does something they should not while using your password, you will get the blame and potentially face disciplinary action.

Remember, e-mails and any other information stored on a computer form legal documents. Be professional at all times and do not compromise patient confidentiality.

Many computers on clinical placements are connected to a trust intranet. Make good use of this as it can be a resource that contains information on wards, departments, policies, clinical guidelines and local events and news.

CLINICAL SKILLS

Each and every clinical skill you are required to learn as a medical student will not be described in detail. However, keep in mind the following advice.

Find out what clinical skills you are expected to become proficient in early on and ensure that you practise them as regularly as possible. Not only will this enable you to pass your exams but you will be a more slick and professional doctor in the long run.

Do not just learn how to perform a clinical test or examination, but also the underlying principles. This will assist you to perform and interpret the results more comprehensively.

The first time you perform a practical skill, such as taking blood from a real patient, it can be very daunting. Venepuncture (taking blood) and cannulation (putting a more permanent needle into a vein, for example for a drip) are skills that you will use again and again as a junior doctor. It is important to practise these as a student as much as you can.

Human instinct makes us avoid doing things we are nervous about, but as a student it is important to overcome these fears and get all the practical experience you can. Most patients are understanding and realise that you need to learn. If you do not feel confident at something then take a doctor along with you so that they can help and give you tips when necessary.

Always say 'yes' when a doctor asks you if you would like to do something practical, such as performing a blood gas (taking blood from an artery), inserting a nasogastric tube (tube that is inserted into the nose and runs to the stomach) or performing a speculum examination (visualising the neck of the womb). If you have never performed the skill before, tell the doctor and they will talk you through the procedure before you go to the patient. Doctors are good at choosing the right kind of patients for you to perform these skills on; for example, they are unlikely to choose nervous patients or those with needle phobias.

Most of all be confident, don't tell the patient you have never put a cannula in before just as you are putting the needle into their skin, and if you do fail, don't be afraid to ask for help. (*Ali Williams, fourth-year medical student, Leeds*)

ETHICS

Medicine is rife with ethical issues. Throughout your training you must demonstrate an appreciation of ethical dilemmas and an ability to be ethically sound in your work. Appreciate the difference between ethics and law: you are required by law to follow certain rules; however, to be a good and appropriate doctor you must also follow ethical guidance. In general, ethical behaviour lies within the law, but this is not necessarily the case. The General Medical Council (GMC) sets out guidance and assesses your performance in accordance to law *and* ethics. Do not disregard ethics as a 'touchy feely' subject, but learn the principles thoroughly to prevent premature cessation of your medical career.

The main points of good ethical practice can be remembered by use of the letters A–F:[5]

➡ autonomy: give the patient choice and encourage them to make decisions
➡ beneficence: do good
➡ confidentiality
➡ do no harm and do not lie

➡ everyone else: you have a duty to society
➡ fairness and justice.

When faced with an ethical problem, try and work through and weigh up factors A–F and determine what is the best, most ethical, course of action. Globally correct answers do not exist for any situation; this is not a topic you can revise and learn the answers to. A good ethical approach includes an appreciation that your job as a doctor involves doing good, not only for your patient, but to the society in which we all live. An illustration of this is breaking confidentiality. Most people understand the concept of confidentiality in doctor–patient relationships and how it 'should not be broken'. However, what about the case in which a pathologically jealous patient has disclosed, to you as a GP, he intends to kill his wife's boss, with whom he thinks she is having an affair? The patient has told you he has the gun in his car and will go straight to the boss's office after leaving his appointment. Do you still have to maintain the husband's confidentiality in order to fulfil your duty to him as the patient? The answer is 'no' if you think his threat is real. You have a duty to break the patient's confidentiality in order to fulfil your role and protect society, or individuals within it.

Potential ethical dilemmas you may face in your medical career are widely variable. However, as a student you need to grasp the concepts of informed consent and confidentiality. Be familiar with published ethical guidance (please note that guidance for England, Scotland, Wales and Northern Ireland can vary from each other). Do not forget, if you are a member of a medical protection organisation you can ring, write to or e-mail them to ask for advice.

> Gillick competence and Fraser guidelines

> Attend or organise an ethical debate.

Informed consent

> Every competent adult has the right to refuse medical treatment, no matter how unwise others may consider the decision.[6]

The purpose of informed consent is not just to prevent litigation; it is crucial for good patient care. Trust is essential for any successful doctor–patient relationship. In order to gain and maintain trust, patient autonomy must be respected. Patients must be free to decide whether or not they undergo treatment or any intervention;

unless in an emergency or if the law prescribes otherwise (e.g. under mental health legislation).

In order to make an informed decision, patients require sufficient, accurate information that they understand. In addition to cultivating trust, informed consent increases co-operation and participation with proposed and agreed management plans.[7]

Patients must consent to your presence as a medical student and your involvement in their care. Importantly, at some point, most medical students have noticed patients being uncomfortable with their presence. Medical students commonly state that there are not adequate systems through which they can obtain consent.[8] This illustrates bad practice that you should not follow blindly.

A major element of informed consent is effective and sufficient communication; not only from doctor to patient but also from patient to doctor. The doctor is responsible for providing information on all aspects of the proposed treatment, procedure, intervention or examination, including the presence of medical students (*see* Box 2.1). Judgement of the required information should include consideration (not assumption) of the patients' beliefs, culture, occupation or any other factor that may affect their personal decision-making process. In addition, patients need to feel comfortable and fulfilled with the information given. They should be encouraged to ask questions, convey what extent of knowledge they wish to gain on their condition and how much they want to be involved in management planning.[7] Obtaining informed consent is a dynamic process. The information required and the needs of the patients will continually change as diagnoses, investigations and management plans progress. Be prepared to repeatedly re-discuss all the areas in Box 2.1. When obtaining consent for your involvement as a medical student, patients must be made aware that their care will not be affected if they refuse your presence.

Box 2.1 Information patients will want (should know) before giving consent[7]

- Diagnosis, including the certainty of that diagnosis or any further investigations necessary to confirm the diagnosis
- Prognosis, with and without treatment
- Treatment and management options, including doing nothing
- Purpose and details of proposed treatment or investigation, including common and/or serious (life-changing) side effects and risks
- Likely benefit of each treatment or management option
- Name of responsible professionals
- Involvement of students or trainees
- Option to change mind: inform patient that this option is available at all times

The two main ways consent can be obtained are *express consent* and *implied consent*.

➡ *Express consent* occurs when patients provide their informed consent in writing or orally. Written consent is preferred (or required) at times. Aside from emergencies, cases requiring written consent include those involving complex treatments or investigations with high or serious risks, procedures for which clinical care is not the primary purpose, where there are potential significant consequences for the patient's life (financial, social, health) and treatment under research.

➡ *Implied consent* is demonstrated when a patient's actions or behaviour implies that they give consent; for example, a patient rolling up their sleeve when you want to take blood. Exercise caution when receiving implied consent, you have no evidence of the patient's full understanding (or lack of it).

To obtain consent you must be suitably trained and qualified, have sufficient knowledge of the proposed treatment or investigation (including risks) and must act in accordance with the guidance on obtaining informed consent laid out by the GMC.[7] As a medical student you will be examining patients, independently performing procedures (e.g. taking blood), taking histories and assisting with procedures. Each of these tasks requires informed consent. Explain all the relevant aspects outlined in Box 2.1 and ensure that the patient knows you are a medical student and the consequences of that. For doctors and medical students alike, performing an examination or procedure without consent amounts to battery or assault. Therefore, if you perform an examination or procedure on a patient it is crucially important, not only for their care but for your career, to clearly document what has been said, what has been done and what consent was given. Medical students are responsible for informing patients that their involvement or examination is to enhance their own medical education, rather than for a direct benefit to the patient.[8] Finally, get to grips with the information given above. Informed consent is an incredibly important topic. It is crucial that you understand the concept fully at this stage to ensure you act ethically and legally in your future practice as a qualified doctor.

Guidance for the general public and clinicians on consent can be found at: www.dh.gov.uk/PolicyAndGuidance/HealthAndSocialCareTopics/Consent/ConsentGeneralInformation/fs/en

Confidentiality

Trust is essential for successful doctor–patient relationships. Not only should patients feel empowered by making their own (well-informed) decisions, they should also trust that whatever is said to the doctor will not be heard by anyone they do not wish to be told. In all but very few occasions, confidentiality is expected of you as a medical student and throughout the rest of your career.

Ensure your patients are aware that you will protect their confidentiality. Without a declaration from you that what they tell you will remain confidential, a patient may not disclose all relevant information, thus making the consultation process harder, a diagnosis less accurate and the management more challenging (even with a declaration of confidentiality patients may still not tell you everything, but that is their prerogative).

It may be even more important for medical students to emphasise their understanding and promise of maintenance of confidentiality. Patients want to be reassured that their story will not be spread around the hospital canteen. Be careful where you leave written records of patients, and where and how you conduct consultations to minimise the chances of inadvertent breaches of confidentiality.

As a medical student, you are likely to discuss a case with doctors in order to learn; inform the patient that you will not discuss their case with anyone not already involved in their care. If you want to recount or present a case formally to people not involved directly with the patient's management it is important that you seek consent of the patient and remove identifying details where possible.

Although there are exceptions to confidentiality that you should be aware of (e.g. when a patient poses a particularly high risk to others), you rarely or never need to break confidentiality as a medical student. If a patient has divulged information

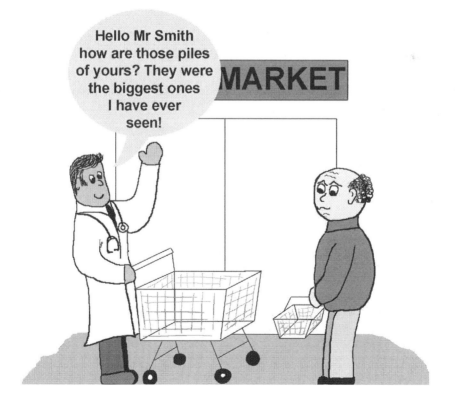

that you think represents a risk to someone else, you can tell the doctors already involved in the patient's care. A patient may tell you something and then ask you not to tell anyone, including the doctors involved in their care. In such cases, or any other you are unsure about, refer to the GMC guidance on confidentiality[9] and/or seek advice from your medical protection organisation, if you are a member.

TIPS FOR SUCCESSFUL CLINICAL EXPERIENCE

> Clinical education must reflect the changing patterns of healthcare and provide experience in a variety of clinical settings.[10]

> We have found that getting on the wards, taking histories and examining patients in pairs is much better than being part of a massive group crowded round the bed with a consultant. Consultant teaching is essential, but you really need to have additional practice, and patients are often happy to help. (*Kate Fraser, fourth-year medical student, Manchester*)

Know your boundaries

Do not do anything you feel inadequately trained to do. This is unethical and unsafe. You will not be disciplined if you refuse to do something; use the opportunity to be taught, shown or supervised doing the procedure again.

Under no circumstances should you initiate, change or stop treatment of a patient under your own instruction or from your own diagnosis. It does not matter how good you think you are: you have not proved your ability until you have graduated.

Do not prescribe medication, request radiological or diagnostic investigations, or order blood for cross-matching. If you want to practise filling out the appropriate request forms, get them countersigned by your supervising doctors. Until you have the experience, training and qualification under your belt, you may expose the patients to unnecessary tests and corresponding risks.

Make sure others know your boundaries

Ensure that patients understand your position, role and, to some extent, lack of qualification. Do not mislead patients into thinking you are a qualified doctor, and clear up any confusion as it arises. This also extends to staff members, who are used to ward doctors changing regularly.

Wear your ID badge at all times and make sure it is clearly visible. Your ID badge will not only inform people that you are allowed to be there but also who you are. The breast pocket area is the preferred location of the badge for others to be able to see it easily without embarrassment.[11] Some healthcare environments will not allow you entry without an ID badge. Do not miss a good learning opportunity because you have lost or forgotten your badge.

Personal care

You are responsible for keeping yourself healthy (mentally and physically) for personal benefit and to protect current or future patients. Eat and sleep adequately and avoid cigarettes and excessive alcohol. Seek prompt help for health problems that you or your friends, family or tutors identify.

Personal care also includes grooming and personal hygiene. Regardless of sterile procedures, no patient wants a grubby student examining them.

NHS occupational health smart cards are being introduced across the UK. Medical students are among the first to be recruited on the smart card system. The cards state who you are, display a picture of you and carry information about your occupational health clearance status. The cards are intended to be an easy way to transfer your occupational health history between your clinical placements or jobs.

What to wear?

You may scoff at this section. 'I am a respectable member of the community and made it through a medical school interview. I think I am quite capable of knowing what I should wear.' But are you? Until now you have probably spent most of your waking hours in jeans, perhaps you even wear a hoodie (!). Now you need to look smart, respectable, comfortable and appropriate for ward life.

> Respondents felt more comfortable talking about their sexual, psychological and more personal matters with physicians who dressed more professionally.[12]

In most circumstances male medical students are not required to wear a suit. However, smart trousers, a shirt and tie are often expected. Please do not try and be 'quirky' with comedy ties. They do not look 'cool' or 'funny' when you are with a doctor who is telling a woman her husband has just died suddenly. If you do wear a tie, be aware that it can dangle; across patients, wounds and bowls of unmentionables. Make sure you tuck it into your shirt or the top of your trousers while you are near patients.

White coats should be clean and pressed. Choose a cool outfit to go underneath as the white coat is often an unwelcome layer in a hot ward or clinic.

General rules include the following.
➡ *Do not wear trainers on clinical placement.* They may be comfortable for a long day on your feet but they give a bad impression. Even if your trainers were the most expensive, sought-after pair in the world, the older ladies you will be attending to will not realise this and will see you as being scruffy.

➥ *Jewellery.* Very little jewellery is appropriate. Big earrings can be dangerous if a young, confused or aggressive patient grabs them. Facial piercings damage a patient's trust and confidence in you. Jewellery can get lost, broken, scratch patients and harbour bacteria, so avoid wearing it.

➥ *Be careful not to wear anything that may offend or be sexually suggestive.* This encompasses clothing that displays slogans, is low-cut, too short or results in a gaping midriff.

➥ *Do not go to a patient wearing your bag or coat.* Even if you are late to a ward round or something interesting happens just as you are leaving. It is really rude and unhygienic.

Be courteous

Use a formal salutation for the patient, e.g. Mrs X, Mr Y, sir, etc., until invited to do otherwise. Patients will often tell you to call them by their first name, but do not assume this is acceptable.

Pull the curtains around the bed when you are taking a history or performing an examination or procedure. Even if not required for dignity, it provides a feeling of privacy (even though everyone is aware that curtains are not soundproof). It will also help you to feel less flustered when you are starting out.

Hospital communication systems

Do not abuse hospital telephones. They are there for work-related communication. Do not use the telephones for your personal calls. This is a misuse of time that should be used for learning and you may be stopping important calls getting through.

Telephones and pagers are the backbone of hospital communication. Patients are spread around many wards, and you may need to visit many departments if you are to experience all that is on offer or want to follow a patient's journey. It is essential that you know how to contact all the people and places that are required. Carry with you a list of important and useful phone or pager numbers. This will be invaluable when you are a doctor; you may as well get into the habit now. Useful numbers to make a note of may include: your main wards (there is often more than one phone number for each ward); junior doctors and registrar pager numbers for your team; X-ray Department; haematology, microbiology, blood bank and biochemistry departments (useful for results, advice and other related queries); theatre (if you are on a surgical team) and the medical school.

Active learning

You will not learn through osmosis while on a ward or at a GP surgery. Seek out interesting cases, patients with 'good signs' and those with complex problems. Get teaching from as many of the doctors as you can. All will have something to offer; they are all more experienced than you.

See as many patients as possible. (Nat Bradbrook, fifth-year medical student, Manchester)

During teaching, answer questions using the correct terminology rather than pointing or using layman's terms. Although you need to practise using lay language for patients, you also need to demonstrate your knowledge to your tutors.

Read up on the day's patients, conditions and experiences in the evening. You will gain much more from your time on placement if you integrate clinical and book work. If you know you are having a teaching session on a particular topic, read up on it the night before. This allows quick confirmation of the basic information and teaching can move on to the more important or interesting aspects of the topic.

Be proactive. Do not wait around for doctors to come and teach you – go and ask them for teaching. A doctor who thinks you are keen is more likely to teach. (Nat Bradbrook, fifth-year medical student, Manchester)

Keep up to date with 'hot topics'. The media often covers medicine-related areas. Make sure you know what is being said to the general public and the supporting or correct facts behind the stories. Patients, consultants or examiners may ask you about such topics. Examples of such are the MMR vaccination and autism, breast cancer treatments and child abuse.

Have fun. Providing you are professional and appropriate at all times your clinical training should be enjoyable. You may feel silly when you get excited about clinical signs or an interesting case, but this serves as proof that you are right to be doing medicine.

LEARNING HOSPITAL LINGO

Perhaps this is the hardest component of a medical degree. The language of medicine does not just include learning long difficult words, but the shortened and slang versions of many phrases, words and expressions. Medics play with speech until it is totally confusing. This section will give you the upper hand when you hit the wards and can understand what is going on. Do note, however, that many of the below are not politically correct, not specific or are medico-legally or ethically unsound. This is a reference for your understanding and not a dictionary of terms to use – it will be your integrity on the line.

Slang words

Medics use slang terms for everyday words. For example, 'tubes' refers to a stethoscope.

'Heartsink' patients are well known among medics. You may think it is a cardiology term for an electromechanical disorder of the heart; the more intelligent may even think it is spelt 'heartsync'. However, the term is used to describe a patient who 'makes your heart sink' when they walk in the room; NEVER write this in someone's notes.

The 'firm' is the group of doctors, or multi-disciplinary team, who work together. It will often include a doctor of each grade. You will be attached to a 'firm' in your clinical years, which means that you are not just attached to the consultant. Make sure you make good use of all members of the firm.

A patient's smoking history is described in terms of a 'pack-year' history. One pack-year is anything that equates to 20 cigarettes a day for one year. This may be 10 cigarettes a day for two years or 40 cigarettes a day for six months. Therefore, a patient who is aged 78 and has been smoking 20 cigarettes a day since the age of 15 years has a 63 pack-year smoking history. Working this out is important as it provides a good estimation of a patient's exposure to cigarette smoke.

Codes

Doctors may use code language while giving you instructions or talking about patients. For example, in the examination setting, if you are asked to examine a patients 'hands' this means, 'please examine this patient's hands, elbows (for rheumatoid nodules and psoriasis) and ears (for signs of gout and psoriasis)'. Similarly, if you are asked to examine a patient's 'chest' you have just been given the instruction to examine the patient's hands, blood pressure, neck, face, thorax, abdomen and legs (in some cases), and listen to the heart and lungs. It is important that you identify the consultants who use these codes and clarify what you are being asked if you are unsure what the real question or request is.

The use of code language while talking about patients is often unique to each consultant. Some examples may include describing a patient's history as 'unfortunate', implying that virtually every system in a patient's body is diseased and that they should have been dead some time ago. Similarly, if a doctor states that family dynamics may require investigation it often implies the diagnosis has a psychological basis, trigger or maintaining factor.

Acronyms

Don't be caught out by the consultant telling you 'this patient has previously had a cabbage'. 'Big deal', you may think, but don't be fooled. It is highly likely, in the medical setting, that the patient has had a coronary artery bypass graft – a CABG. This is a big operation in which the blocked arteries around the heart are replaced, often with veins from the patient's leg.

Medics are well known for their acronyms, some are useful to know when starting your clinical placements in order to decipher medical notes (*see* Box 2.2). However, be aware that in medico-legal terms acronyms are not acceptable nor are they recommended as they can lead to potentially harmful misunderstandings.

Box 2.2 Acronyms you may see in clinical notes
- JACCOL (jaundice, anaemia, clubbing, cyanosis, oedema, lymphadenopathy)
- LOC (loss of consciousness)
- NOF (neck of femur)
- ORIF (open reduction and internal fixation)
- POP (plaster of Paris)
- SOB (short of breath)
- TOE (transoesophageal echocardiography)

Abbreviations

Ward rounds are busy and may lead to information being written down as quickly as possible. Abbreviations become as natural to write as your name. However, writing abbreviations leads to miscommunication or even lack of communication if the reader deciphers the author's notes incorrectly. Therefore this is not a lesson of which abbreviations to use when, but rather to assist you, as the reader of clinical notes, to understand what has been written. Box 2.3 demonstrates a few common abbreviations.

Box 2.3 Abbreviations you may read in clinical notes
- ° (not present, e.g. °pain = 'no pain')
- ∴ (therefore)
- # (fracture, or bleep number)
- C/O (complaining of)
- F/U (follow up)
- LFT (liver function test) (blood test)
- Imp (impression)
- I/P (inpatient)
- Ix (investigations)
- Obs (observations: blood pressure, pulse, respiratory rate, temperature)
- O/D (overdose or outpatient department)
- Rx (treatment)
- Sats (oxygen saturation levels in the blood)
- TFT (thyroid function test) (blood test)
- U&E (urea and electrolytes) (blood test)

ANSWER TEMPLATES FOR CLINICAL QUESTIONS

It is frustrating when you know all the answers but nobody bothers asking you the questions.[2]

On many occasions, questions you are asked in the clinical setting may be answered by use of a range of generic templates. It is highly advisable to learn these and use them when learning and recalling information. Using the templates given below (or your own) ensures that your answers and thoughts are logical, systematic and less likely to be incomplete. Michael Barrie has written a book, *The Surgeon's Rhyme: a memoir,*[2] which, in addition to illustrating his medical career, demonstrates the usefulness of having a template on which to hang answers to many questions. By learning the templates below, you will not have to remember lists of information but will be able to work out the answer.

➡ *What would you do if a patient presented with X?* Always, before you say anything else, state 'I would take a full history and perform a thorough examination' – make sure you know what you would examine (when appropriate).

➡ *What is the general approach to diagnosis?* Full history, examination and investigations.

➡ *What investigations would you perform on this patient?* This clearly depends on what is wrong with the patient and whether investigations are appropriate. However, the general rule is to start simple, safe, cheap and basic before progressing to more sophisticated, rationed and invasive procedures. What follows is an example and is not exhaustive. Simple tests to start with include blood, urine, drain fluid, sputum or other samples for biochemistry, haematology, culture or cytology. Once you feel confident you have covered these, move on to relatively simple imaging techniques (ultrasound, plain X-ray) before moving on to more sophisticated (e.g. CT scans, MRI scans) or invasive (e.g. biopsy, endoscopy, laparoscopy) investigations which carry a risk to the patient's health and life. Obviously there are exceptions so ensure you read local and national guidelines and follow the advice of senior colleagues.

➡ *Tell me about condition X?* The template of this answer is called the 'disease profile'. Describe the condition taking into account all aspects of a disease in a systematic way. A conventional way of doing this is shown in Box 2.4.

Box 2.4 Structure of a disease profile
- Incidence and epidemiology (how many and who the disease affects)
- Aetiology (the factors causing the disease)
- Pathogenesis (the processes by which the disease develops)
- Pathological features (abnormalities – seen within the body, system or tissues – resulting from the disease)
- Clinical features (symptoms and signs)
- Complications
- Treatment (investigations and management)
- Prognosis, with and without treatment

➡ *What are the causes of condition X?* On being asked this question you will often immediately think of rare, humorous or exciting causes; not necessarily the most common or important. Therefore you need a template on which to structure your answer based on the mechanisms by which the disease (or symptom) arises; a 'surgical sieve' (*see* Box 2.5; *see also The Medical Student's Survival Guide 1: the early years*).

Box 2.5 Pathological categories comprising a 'surgical sieve'
- **Iatrogenic (caused by the actions of the medical profession)**
- **Neoplastic (benign or malignant)**
- **Vascular (including blood and heart)**
- **Endocrine**
- **Structural or mechanical**
- **Trauma or accident**
- **Inflammatory**
- **Genetic or congenital**
- **Autoimmune**
- **Toxic**
- **Infective**
- **Old age or degenerative**
- **Nutritional or metabolic**
- **Spontaneous or idiopathic**

➡ *What are the causes of obstruction of a tube* (e.g. of the bowel, ureters (kidneys to bladder), bronchi (airways in the lungs))? Intraluminal (within the tube), such as growths, stones or foreign bodies; within the wall, such as narrowing caused by scar tissue or thickening of the wall; external compression; growths or scar tissue arising from structures around the outside of the tube.

➡ *What are the complications of procedure X?* Discuss complications in terms of immediate, short-term and long-term complications. Always consider bleeding and infection for all invasive procedures and mention complications of general anaesthetics for relevant surgery.

➡ *How would you counsel a patient for a diagnostic or screening test?* This template may be adapted to cover tests such as an HIV test right through to pre-natal screening tests. Once you have performed preliminary steps such as introduction and consent, ensure you explicitly state that confidentiality will be maintained. Some diagnostic tests are sensitive and have huge repercussions for patients; they must feel confident in you. Ask why the patient thinks they need the test. Ask them to discuss with you the risks they feel they (or the baby) have. You may take this opportunity to then qualify their perceived risks and discuss other risk factors for the condition you will be testing or screening for. Identify what the patient understands is involved in the test and what the results mean. Clarify any misconceptions the patient has and ensure they understand exactly what is involved. Discuss the advantages and disadvantages of having the test, including the likelihood of incorrect results. Ask what the patient thinks they will do if the test is positive or negative and the implications of a positive or negative test. Provide details of support should the results be unfavourable. Ensure the patient has adequate support during decision-making about the test and during the interim period before the results are known. Summarise what you have spoken about with the patient and clearly ask them whether they still want the test. Gain consent and record what has been said and the consent in the patient's notes.

HOW TO WEAR A STETHOSCOPE

To the unsuspecting, wearing a stethoscope could not be more easy. You pick it up, place it around your neck and – hey presto – you look like you know what you are doing and people think you are a doctor. However, incorrect placement of the stethoscope can result in pain and danger. The illustration below demonstrates the best way to wear your stethoscope! Traditionally, wearing your stethoscope around your neck is considered unprofessional. In exam situations you may be required to hold your stethoscope in your hand.

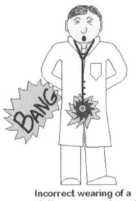

Incorrect wearing of a stethoscope can be painful....

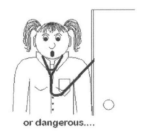

or dangerous....

get it right and stay happy!!!!

FURTHER READING

Beasley R, Robinson G, Aldington S. From medical student to junior doctor: accepting the responsibility of informed consent. *StudentBMJ*. 2006; **14**: 94–6. (This article contains an excellent summary of the principles of consent, example cases to test your understanding and further references.)

British Medical Association. *Consent Tool Kit*. London: British Medical Association; 2003. (Excellent resource that details the answers to many, commonly encountered questions regarding consent in various situations.)

General Medical Council. *Withholding and Withdrawing Life-prolonging Treatments: good practice in decision making*. London: General Medical Council; 2002.

Modra L. The fashion doctor. *StudentBMJ*. 2006; **14**: 302–3.

CHAPTER 3

Talking with patients and colleagues

Although only practice and experience can assist the unsure to communicate effectively with patients and colleagues this chapter will provide an insight into the importance of this skill as well as tips for beginners and common pitfalls.

The General Medical Council (GMC) includes 'the ability to communicate clearly' as one of the two fundamental skills required for the practice of medicine.[1] Poor and inappropriate communication creates anxiety for you and your patients and it is the greatest source of patient dissatisfaction.[2] Poor communication with colleagues, especially when handing over care, results in a danger to patients' health and safety.[3] Many medical students struggle with this important skill. If you are one of these students, all is not lost. It is increasingly recognised that communication skills are not solely inherent but can be taught, learned and retained.[4]

THE IMPORTANCE OF LEARNING GOOD COMMUNICATION

> Most people tell you that the most important qualities a doctor can have are good communication skills and an efficient and pleasant doctor-patient relationship. These are the hardest things to learn and perfect. But, being able to initiate a consultation, even if you cannot reach a diagnosis, gives you a buzz and a confidence that will carry the rest of your clinical skills. (*Zoe Cowan, first-year medical student, Leicester*)

Imagine you are admitted to hospital. You do not know what is wrong with you but you have been feeling lousy for a while. Aches and pains have stopped you from getting a good night's sleep for a number of weeks; fever is muddling your thought processes and, just when you want to crawl into a corner and hide, you are thrust into a building in which you are expected to live, eat and (try to) sleep with a bunch of strangers. Every morning doctors, nurses and young people in white coats come to you and mumble something about an '*itis*' or an '*ology*' (and it is hoped not an '*oma*') and then leave again. You did not get a chance to ask the question you have been trying to ask since you arrived and you still do not know when you can go home or why they are sticking a needle in you everyday.

Life in hospital can be pretty miserable, without it being made worse by poor communication. It is your duty as a doctor, medical student or any other healthcare professional, to make your patient's stay as easy as possible. Even attending an outpatient department, GP surgery or other healthcare consultation is daunting. The most effective way of reducing fear, anxiety and even hostility is to ensure that communication is accurate, understandable and relevant.

Medical school graduates must 'communicate clearly, sensitively and accurately' with patients, their friends and family and all healthcare colleagues.[5] You must identify the views, feelings, opinions and beliefs of these individuals. Communication does not always occur through speech. Although you are not expected to learn sign language, for example, be aware that various channels of communication exist, and think how you can work with interpreters.

Insufficient or difficult communication with colleagues not only presents a danger to yourself and your patients, it can increase everybody's workload. Each team member may look up the same test results or ask patients identical questions. Learn to speak up when it is appropriate and to pipe down when someone more 'clued up' is talking. Communication with colleagues includes written communication. Document what you have done, what you are (not) going to do and why.

> Be aware of alternative methods of communication, e.g. Deafblind Manual and British Sign Language

Medical schools provide you opportunity to practise your communication skills using various methods, devices and situations. Some situations are particularly challenging, for example breaking bad news or communication with difficult individuals (see Chapter 14) and communication with a patient who knows little English. Learn how to alter your communication style to adapt to these situations by observing others; be proactive and observe as many different situations as appropriate.

THE DIFFERENCE BETWEEN MEN AND WOMEN

It is consistently recognised that women perform better at communication skills than men. Female doctors' consultations are often more likely to be conversational, involve the patients and (although consultations are longer) address psychosocial issues.[4] Women also hold a more positive attitude towards communication skills training.[4] Therefore, if you do not hold communication skills training in high regard, perhaps you should change your mind. Undertake the training from a positive frame of mind and you may become a better communicator.

HOW TO LEARN COMMUNICATION SKILLS

> The better doctors communicate with their patients, the fewer number of complaints and claims against them. Conversely, doctors who relate poorly to their patients attract higher than average complaints and claims, regardless of their technical ability.[6]

Practise

There is no substitute for communication practise in real settings. By the time you graduate, you should have refined communication skills and experience of the following situations.

➡ Taking informed consent (Chapter 2).
➡ Ensuring the patient understands confidentiality (Chapter 2).
➡ Taking a history from a patient and their relatives/carers (Chapter 4).
➡ Negotiation with colleagues.
➡ Resolving conflict.
➡ Assertiveness.
➡ Negotiation of medical management, including two-way communication covering patient ideas, concerns and expectations; also learn how to offer solutions and follow-up.
➡ 'Do not resuscitate' orders, not necessarily discussing this with patients/family but build your confidence in being involved in such discussions with colleagues.
➡ Breaking bad news.

Spend as much time as you can in wards, clinics and GP surgeries. Some lonely or nervous patients enjoy 'just having a chat'. Take advantage of the time that medical students have to just chat about everyday things with patients. This simple task will build your confidence and experience of communicating with, for example, older patients, those who are deaf and those who speak a different language. Some talkative patients will force you into practising the art of closing or leading a conversation: skills that are invaluable when your time is pressured.

Progression through medical school carries a risk of reduction in communication skills. Sometimes senior medical students focus on diagnosing the patient rather more than they concentrate on the doctor–patient relationship and communication skills.[4] Remember to concentrate on your communication skills just as much as the history you are taking.

> I really enjoyed the communications skills sessions which used simulated patients (actors) to practise on. Early sessions were designed to help you to develop history-taking skills. There was an option for a 'pause button',

where you could ask advice from fellow students when you were stuck. You also received feedback from the actor and your tutor. (*Imran Sajid, fourth-year medical student, Manchester*)

Medical school communication sessions

Medical school communication sessions using simulated patients (trained actors) allow you to practise communication techniques and skills in difficult situations without risking the mental health of your patients! The first time you have to communicate with upset or angry patients is very daunting. Simulated patients and medical school communication skills sessions allow you to practise, ask for direction or assistance and rewind conversations until you manage them well.

Medical students sometimes do their utmost to avoid communication skills sessions. However, feedback and tips from the simulated patients, tutors and your classmates can be invaluable. In addition, communication skills training results in better problem diagnosis during interviews with patients.[4]

Other techniques used by medical schools to improve your communication skills involve video recordings of consultations with a simulated patient. You and your class then watch and critically evaluate how you did. This allows step-by-step analysis of the consultation and exact assessment of what worked and what did not.

External help
Professional Medical Education

For those of you who might feel overwhelmed, Professional Medical Education (PME) (www.freefees.co.uk) can teach you how to be assertive on their assertiveness and communication skills courses. Not sure how to deal with nurses or other allied health professionals? Their courses will assist you to become a confident, polite and well-spoken doctor.

BREAKING BAD NEWS

Breaking bad news is one of the most unpleasant aspects of being a medic. 'Bad news' may make you think of terminal diagnoses; however, bad news comes in many forms and differs between patients.

Think about the following (simplistic) example: two men are in theatre recovery after amputation of a leg. The first man wakes up and is told he has had his leg amputated; he cannot remember the car accident he was in, his dreams of being a professional footballer are shattered and he is devastated. The second man wakes up soon afterwards, is told the same news and is delighted. Surely this is not a normal response? What if the second patient had been in severe pain from an ischaemic leg (not enough blood getting to the tissues)? Loss of this painful limb results in total relief, it is no wonder he was delighted, he will be able to sleep in a bed again.

Although the above example is grossly simplistic (and unrealistic in terms of consent), it illustrates the point that a piece of news may be good or bad depending on the situation in which it is given. The first important point to learn for breaking bad news is to know when you will be breaking bad news.

Never break bad news unless you have observed and practised the skill. Once you are experienced enough to break bad news, follow these simple steps before you approach the patient and family.

➡ Gather all available information.
➡ Understand all test results and their significance. If a test result shows a 'likely' diagnosis this is different to a 'definite' diagnosis. Appreciate this and decide how appropriate it is to tell the patient or family a 'likely' diagnosis.
➡ Think about the likely or definite management plan.

Models of how to break bad news may vary; however, a well-known technique is the SPIKES model:[7]

➡ *Setting*: make sure the setting is appropriate and private (e.g. you are not in a busy corridor) and ensure you have people with you to provide support to you (colleagues) and the patient (relatives, friends and nurses) if required. Turn your bleep and mobile phone off. Ensure there are some tissues to hand.
➡ *Perception*: assess the patient's understanding of the situation to date. Ask what they know already, what has happened and what they have been told. You can also ask what they think is going on.
➡ *Invitation*: ask the patient if they would like you to give them more information. You can ask if they would like to know everything, providing them with control of how much information they receive.

> Would you like me to go through your test results with you?

➡ *Knowledge*: provide information in small chunks and use simple but accurate language. Summarise what has happened up to the present day. Use warning shots (*see below*) before the actual information is given. Once the information is given, pause. Give the patient time to ponder what has been said. Provide enough time for (and invite) questions. Regularly clarify the patient's understanding.

> It must be a shock

➡ *Empathy and emotions*: You cannot know what it feels like for the recipient every time you break bad news. However, you can show them that you understand their distress and you should comfort them in an appropriate way.

> I know this is not what you wanted to hear

➡ *Strategy and summary*: Never drop the patient or relatives into the depths of despair and then abandon them. Try and end the bad news with a glimmer of realistic hope, or at least the way forward from now. Suggest management plans (e.g. pain relief, anti-sickness medication, treatment options, post-death procedures), the offer of support from nurses, other organisations (e.g. charities) that may be of assistance and your return in a specified time period to answer questions that may arise.

'Warning shots' are used throughout the initial break-ing bad news process. Warning shots are statements that imply bad news is coming but do not give the information. They may be simplified medical or everyday phrases such as 'I am afraid'. Warning shots may increase in intensity throughout the invitation and knowledge stages of SPIKES, for example:

> Is this what you feared?

- ➡ warning shot 1: 'We have got your test results back which have shown an abnormality'
- ➡ warning shot 2: 'The abnormality we have found may be serious'
- ➡ warning shot 3: 'The test has shown a growth . . .'
- ➡ information: 'The growth is a type of cancer.'

After you have broken bad news, or witnessed the process, reflect on the process. What went well? What did not? Was the SPIKES model used? Which phrases were effective? Did the patient fully understand what was said? What state did you leave the recipient in? How do you feel? If you have found the whole process tough, talk to a friend or colleague, especially those who were present when the bad news was broken. Gain feedback on how others thought it went. Praise each other for completing such an unpleasant task.

> Ask to observe different doctors breaking bad news. Look at the different approaches, what works and what does not.

PHRASES MEDICS USE WHICH CAUSE CONFUSION

Medical jargon is best avoided when possible. Medical students are not fully comprehensive in the art of speaking 'medical' even at graduation. However, certain words and phrases used in medicine, although not medical words *per se*, can result in misunderstanding and confusion in professionals and patients alike.

- ➡ *Negative and positive results.* Negative is sometimes mistakenly interpreted as meaning bad (there is a disease present, something is wrong, what they were testing for was there) and positive as good (i.e. they are not ill, the disease being tested for is not present).

➥ *False-positive and false-negative.* A false-positive result occurs when a test has indicated a condition or risk is present when it is not. A false-negative result occurs when tests indicate the condition or risk is not present when it is.

➥ *Hyper- and hypo-.* Hyper = high or too much; hypo = low or too little.

➥ *Cancer described as progressing.* Do not believe this means the cancer is getting better and smaller or disappearing. It is the total opposite (i.e. the cancer is getting worse or spreading).

➥ *Diagnostic and screening tests.* Screening tests are not diagnostic. Screening tests simply assess the risk or likelihood of a condition being present. They do not indicate a condition is definitely present. A diagnostic test is one that identifies whether the disease or condition is present or not. Both screening and diagnostic tests can be subject to false-positive and false-negative results (*see above*) and are reliant on the specificity and sensitivity of the test method (*see below*).

➥ *Specificity and sensitivity.* These terms describe the usefulness of tests or screening. If a test or screening programme is sensitive, it will pick out most or all the positive results that are present within the sample. For example, a sensitive test for diabetes will find all the patients tested with high blood sugar to have high blood sugar. The specificity of a test or screening programme describes, out of the patients found to have the trait being tested for, how many have the disease or condition the test or screening was designed to detect. For example, testing the urine for glucose will identify patients with diabetes but also those with a low renal glucose threshold; thus the specificity of urine glucose testing as a way of detecting diabetes is low.

➥ *Tumour.* Be very careful when using the word 'tumour'. Members of the public may think this is synonymous with cancer. However the term 'tumour' actually means a mass of abnormally growing cells, this can be benign (non-cancerous) or malignant (cancerous). If you use the word 'tumour' for a benign mass make sure you clearly state this.

➥ *Stage and grade of cancer.* Staging simply means how far a cancer has spread. Grading cancer describes how abnormal or malignant the cancerous cells are.

➥ *Inter- and intra-.* These prefixes are often used interchangeably and should not be. 'Inter-' means between and 'intra-' means on the inside. For example, *inter*cellular processes = processes occurring from cell-to-cell interaction; *intra*cellular processes = processes occurring within the cell.

PATIENTS DO NOT ALWAYS SAY WHAT THEY MEAN

Not only do medics create confusion by using words that patients do not understand, patients can be equally confusing (and amusing) when they attempting to indulge in 'medic speak'. Below is the beginner's guide to understanding the laypersons' medical language.

➡ *Asteroids*: an inventive, imaginative and accurate description of steroids. An elderly lady devised this term after undergoing a dramatic recovery solely attributed to these drugs.

➡ *Cafetiere*: the astute may realise that patients are not referring to their ground coffee infusion device but a catheter, an indwelling, bladder draining device.

➡ *Calpol*: older patients may ask for this paediatric paracetamol-containing medication, but is this really what they want? Patients have asked for this when they actually meant the indigestion remedy Gaviscon.

➡ *Glucose*: this sugary substance has been used to describe mucous; the importance of this mistake occurs mainly in cooking!

➡ *Lucozade*: depending on the situation this has been known to translate to lactulose. Be sure to alleviate this confusion, you do not want patients drinking bottles of the osmotic laxative.

➡ *Palpations*: patients rarely report the feeling that they are being touched or physically examined. If this does happen, consider the possibility that they are experiencing palpitations, the awareness of their own heartbeat.

➡ *Prostrate*: it would appear that many older gentlemen have increasing difficulties in lying face down, causing them to require trips to the toilet at night to urinate. It does not take a genius to work out that such people are referring to their prostate gland.

PATIENTS ARE NOT ALWAYS SAYING WHAT YOU THINK THEY ARE

There are some words used in day-to-day life that are indicative of certain conditions. In general conversations the exact meaning of such words is irrelevant, however in medicine such words need to be specifically defined by the patient and yourself to ensure you are talking about the same thing. Below are a few examples.

➡ *Chronic*: pain is often referred to as chronic. Medics generally apply the term 'chronic' to the length of time something has been present (unless you are thinking of inflammation –let's forget about that here). Patients often use 'chronic' to describe bad or severe pain.

➡ *Diarrhoea*: this term may describe the passing of one lot of 'loose stool' per day through to an explosive expulsion of large amounts of faecal matter occurring up to 30 times a day. It is immediately apparent that such detail needs to be clarified not only for diagnostic reasons but also when assessing the need for fluid resuscitation and further management.

➡ *Dizziness*: a number of perceptions can be described as dizziness; from light-headedness that accompanies a high temperature, to the feeling that the room is spinning due to alcohol intoxication. If a patient says they have been dizzy ALWAYS ask them to describe this further.

➡ *Palpitations*: palpitations may describe the fluttering feeling of excitement or anxiety through to the experience of missed heartbeats or forceful thumping in the chest. If a patient complains of palpitations ask them to describe exactly what they experience. You could also ask them to tap the sensation out for you.

➡ *Tired*: tiredness is a common complaint. However, there is a big difference between the patient who generally feels lethargic, one who is falling asleep regularly, regardless of where they are, and someone whose muscles have become weak. Make sure you really understand what type of 'tiredness' the patient is referring to.

PATIENCE WITH PATIENTS

Communication is not always easy, and patience is required to obtain a true understanding of a situation. Past medical students have made patients cry because they have become irritated by the patient's inability to answer questions in an 'acceptable' way. This demonstrates misplaced negativity onto the patient from the medical student, who is actually irritated because they cannot think of another way of asking the question.

Patients are not healthcare professions and do not know what information is important (or not). They may state many symptoms that are insignificant to your medical mind, but which may be causing great concern to the patient. Observe how doctors politely move patients on from the less important symptoms while also validating their concerns.

Patients cannot always give the information you require. Tablets may be listed only by colour, shape and size. They believe this is useful information, so do not belittle them. Try asking what they believe the tablet is for. Similarly, patients do not always remember the timescale of their problems: 'It has been going on a while'. More detail is sometimes necessary so help the patient answer your question without putting words in their mouth: 'Has it been happening for days, weeks or months?' For longer periods of time use year landmarks, such as 'Did you have the headache last Christmas?'

CHILDREN

Children may be scared or overexcited when they are ill. Ensure your approach is appropriate. To the scared child, talk in a calm voice, smiling when appropriate and directing questions at both the child and the parent. Taking off your white coat makes you look less intimidating. Speak to the child in a way they can understand and explain everything before you do it. However, providing you have the parent's or carer's permission, do not ask a young child permission to examine them, their likely answer is 'no', especially if they are scared of you: try saying 'I am going to listen to your front now'.

Young children may be shy and intimidated by strangers. In these cases, no amount of discussion of the latest cartoon character or play will engage the child enough to let you examine them. However, if you build good rapport with the parents it can indicate to the child that you are a good person and they may allow you to examine them. Other tricks include letting the child play with your stethoscope while taking a history.

Overexcited children are often amusing. Try not to laugh, this encourages them and just makes matters a whole lot worse! Remain friendly but calm, and whatever you do never mention the word 'tickle' when examining the child; you will no longer be able to touch them without them wriggling, pulling away or screaming with excitement!

GENERAL TIPS TO GET YOU ONE STEP AHEAD

Effective communication is reliant on your ability to adapt and use the appropriate communication channels, language and people. However, a few tips will ease your rocky road to success.

Building rapport is not a generic process. Every patient is different; some may be open to medical students speaking to them for social and/or educational reasons. Others may be shy, anxious or do not want to speak to you. Get down to the patient's eye level (bending your knees, not your back) to avoid appearing dominating and to make the conversation more private. Beware of barging in with the same opening lines every time; you need to adapt your approach to each patient.

Do not interrupt. Sounds obvious? Many healthcare professionals limit the available information by interrupting too early. Many patients, when asked to describe their problem(s), can talk for a good two minutes. However, the average time they are given to speak is 22 seconds.[8] Stay silent, even if there is a slight pause, to make sure your patient has really finished. If you have to speak, encourage the patient to say more: 'Tell me more about . . .' or 'Go on'. Be wary of using the term 'OK'; depending on your tone this can sound quite dismissive.

Use communication with older patients to learn about the history of the local area. This can be helpful in the future, not just for management issues but for initiating conversation with other patients. Some hospital wards are in the same buildings as tuberculosis patients were sent to die many years ago. Older patients who know this and are placed in these wards can become quite distressed at the association. Similarly, knowing the industrial history of an area may alert you to the greater possibility of occupational diseases.

Not all old patients are deaf, but many are a bit! Do not shout at every patient over the age of 60 on the presumption they are hard of hearing. This can sound patronising and is unpleasant to those for whom it is not required. Start by speaking clearly and confidently, you will know very quickly if you are not speaking loud enough for the patient to hear you.

Always ensure two-way understanding. Patients often like to please. Many will nod and agree as you talk to them. However, a proportion will not have understood a word you have said. Continuously check their understanding without being patronising. Equally, ensure you understand what they are describing or saying. Regularly recap what has been said and what you have understood and check with the patient for accuracy and missing information.

> What do you understand from what I have just said?

Watch the patient as you are talking to them and respond to any non-verbal messages they are broadcasting. Topics within medicine are often personal and sometimes embarrassing, worrying or upsetting. Watch for your patients beginning to appear uncomfortable? If this happens, ask them why, stop your questioning or ask their permission to continue. If they are becoming upset, acknowledge this, offer them a tissue and some comfort, for example just a hand on their hand can be very reassuring. Do not plough on through your line of questioning with no regard for your patient's feelings; you will lose rapport and limit your history.

Do not be scared to say you do not know something. Be aware of the balance between not giving your patients confidence in you and misleading them with false certainty. If you do not know what is going on, confidently say this and explain the processes you are using to find out. Patients will appreciate your honesty.

Get someone to fill you in on the local dialect. There are certain areas around the UK which have their own local dialect that is totally different to the language in which symptoms are described in textbooks. This can make history-taking quite difficult, so ask doctors what words they have come across if you are new to the local area. Not only will you have a giggle, this prior investigation will assist your communication with patients in the forthcoming years.

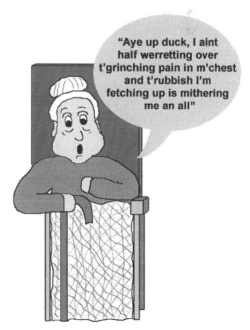

"Aye up duck, I aint half werretting over t'grinching pain in m'chest and t'rubbish I'm fetching up is mithering me an all"

FURTHER READING

Hastings AM, McKinley RK, Fraser RC. Strengths and weaknesses in the consultation skills of senior medical students: identification, enhancement and curricular change. *Med Educ.* 2006; **40**: 437–43.

CHAPTER 4

History-taking

> By cross questioning, the physician would ascertain the symptoms . . . establish the nature of the disease, frame a diagnosis and formulate a regimen.[1]

Medical history-taking is one of the first clinical skills medical students are taught. A good history provides the diagnosis or differential diagnoses in four out of five cases.[2] All medical school graduates are expected to be competent in effectively taking a full medical history.[3] Read Chapter 3 for tips on talking with patients before you begin to learn how to take a history.

You are unlikely to get through you first clinical year without hearing 'There is no such thing as a poor historian, just a poor history taker.' This is true to a great extent. You have to learn the topics you need information on and the different ways of obtaining that information. Take the example below. (The patient has presented with unusual symptoms and the doctor is considering a tropical illness.)

⮕ **Doctor: Have you been abroad recently?**

⮕ **Patient: No**

⮕ **Doctor: Have you been on holiday?**

⮕ **Patient: No**

⮕ **Doctor: Have you been on a plane in the last year?**

⮕ **Patient: Yes, the wife and I went to Africa last month**

This is an extreme, but true, example highlighting the need to phrase questions appropriately to the patient's age, education, culture, language and mental state. Some patients will have no idea what you mean when you ask them 'When did you last open your bowels?' Make sure you can rephrase such questions without causing offence. Only a minority of patients are 'poor historians'. These mainly include those with altered cognitive processes (e.g. through dementia) or those with low IQ. In such cases, learn to elicit a medical history from friends, relatives or other third-party members.

The best places to practise your history-taking skills are in clinics or on the wards. Ask for patients who will give an interesting history. Ward and clinic staff members are usually pretty good at directing you to willing and appropriate patients.

When you are learning how to take a history do not look at the patient's clinical notes before you have spoken to them. If you read the notes the educational benefit of this exercise will be reduced as you (subconsciously) close your questioning around the provisional diagnosis. The notes may also be inaccurate because patients' accounts and stories change. Such changing of the patient's history is frustrating throughout your career; you think you have taken a thorough history only to witness your consultant asking the same questions and getting completely different answers. There are a number of theories on why this change happens (some depend on cynicism, that is, lying patients, malingerers, etc.); the most likely explanation is that the initial questioning triggered the patient to think in more depth after you left. In the time between the first and second consultation a more accurate memory may have been prompted.

HOW TO DO IT

> 'If you listen carefully to the patient they will tell you the diagnosis' (*Sir William Osler*)[4]

How may you gain information from a patient? Visual and physical signs, obtained by examination of a patient (*see* Chapter 5), can be useful but the majority of information about a patient is obtained through verbal communication. Relevant and useful information can be obtained by careful and appropriate questioning. This may sound obvious, but have you ever thought about the different types of questions that exist? The type, quality and reliability of information gained by questioning a patient (carer, friend or relative) are dependent on how you ask the question in the first place.

Questions

There are three major types of questions used in history-taking:

➡ *Closed question*: a question that only gives a limited choice of answer, such as 'yes' or 'no'. For example *'Do you have pain?'*

➡ *Open question*: a question that can be answered freely, with as much or as little information as the responder wants to give. For example *'What is troubling you at the moment?'*

➡ *Probing questions*: these are more direct questions than open questions, as they are based on information already obtained but allow a free response. For example *'In what way does your leg pain affect your daily living?'*

Where possible, ask open questions, especially at the start of the history. This makes it easier for patients to give accurate answers. Do not ask leading questions, for example 'You don't have pain do you?' Patients like to please. They may answer the questions incorrectly because they think it is what you want to hear.

The timing of your questions is important. Multiple questions in one breath confuse patients and result in missed answers. You will feel like you are saving time but your history will not be as thorough.

If you rush in with personal, embarrassing or private questions, you are likely to lose your patient's respect, rapport and confidence. A patient usually will not want to talk to you about their sex life just seconds after learning your name. To ensure optimum timing, use the patient's previous answers as a hook on which to hang your next question. For example, when wanting to ask a diabetic patient about impotence, the patient may raise the topic of marital problems during the preliminary history. You may then ask him to explain the marital problems in more depth. You will gain useful information from and appear interested to the patient by listening to and furthering what they are saying.

Templates

Medical and surgical histories follow a general template (*see* Box 4.1). Using a general template reduces the risk that you will miss significant areas of the patient's history. Box 4.1 can be adapted for problems affecting any system of the body. Think if the questions are relevant before you ask them: do not just reel off the list. Add on system-specific questions that must be asked.

Box 4.1 General history template

- Presenting complaint (PC)
- History of presenting complaint (HPC)
- Past medical history (PMH) (significant past diseases/illnesses, surgery, including complications, trauma)
- Drug history (DH) (now and past, prescribed and over-the-counter (OTC), allergies)
- Family history (FH) (close family is most important – parents, siblings and children – grandparents can also be of use; however, details of cousins and aunties or uncles are rarely required)
- Social history (SH) (smoking, alcohol, drugs, accommodation and living arrangements, marital status, baseline functioning, occupation, pets and hobbies)
- Systems review (SR) (cardiovascular system (CVS), respiratory system (RS), gastrointestinal system (GI), nervous system (NS), musculoskeletal system (MSS), genitourinary system (GUS))

Before you start taking the history gain consent from the patient. Introduce yourself to the patient, stating your name and that you are a medical student. Confirm the name of the patient and ask them what they would like to be called. If anybody is with the patient, ask who they are, their relationship to the patient and if the patient is happy for them to stay in the room. State why you are taking the patient's history and what you are going to do with the information gained. Only then do you ask if it is OK to continue with the history. As a medical student taking a history for practice, you can come back another time. It is nice to elicit whether you are interrupting anything, for example a patient with their visitor if the visitor is paying for parking.

The easier the opening questions the better. You have a chance to calm your nerves and the patient has a chance to gauge you; whether they like your manner and how much they want to tell you. Start with questions such as age, handedness (if taking a neurological history), number of pregnancies (for obstetrics history) and occupation. By the time you have run through these opening questions, rapport with the patient should be developing.

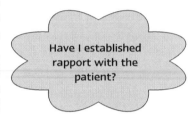

Have I established rapport with the patient?

Presenting complaint

Ask why the patient has come for advice; the 'presenting complaint' (PC). There are a number of ways of approaching this; however, 'Why are you here?' can sound rude. Phrases such as 'What problem has brought you here today?', 'What is troubling you at the moment?' or 'Why has your GP sent you?' may be more appropriate. Patients may have various presenting complaints. This presents a problem to the new clinical student who will list them all. For patients with lists of multiple problems, refine your history in the following ways.

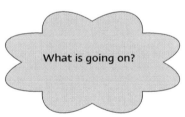

What is going on?

➡ Learn 'red flag' symptoms, that is, those symptoms that indicate a serious disease process is going on. For example, if a patient is complaining of gastrointestinal (GI) symptoms you should elicit whether any GI red flag symptoms are present. Such red flags may include significant weight loss, sudden onset of symptoms, inability to swallow or significant change in bowel habit. If you know what symptoms are 'red flag' you can concentrate on them.

➡ Determine which symptom or problem is the most troubling for the patient. It is these troublesome symptoms that reduce a patient's quality of life the most.

History of the presenting complaint

Once you have established the presenting complaint(s), identify the precise details of the current problem(s): the 'history of the presenting complaint(s)' (HPC). A well-described acronym, SOCRATES, can be used to remember the features of the complaint you should try and determine (*see* Box 4.2). SOCRATES is best used to elicit the features of pain; however, it is useful for many symptoms.

It can be fruitful to ask why a patient has decided to consult a doctor about their problem at that time. Try and discover any reasons for delayed presentation. Ask the patient what they think the problem is and/or if they have known anyone else with similar symptoms. Although some patients object to being asked what they think is going on, 'You tell me, you are the expert', it is important to find out the patient's ideas and concerns. If a patient has consulted with a vague symptom you may wish to tell them that nothing is wrong and send them on their way. However, the patient may be petrified they have cancer. If you do not ask them what they think is wrong you will never discover this. With knowledge of their concern, appropriate reassurance may be given and patient satisfaction will be improved.

Finally, no history of the presenting complaint is complete until you have discovered the effects of the problem on the patient's activities of daily living. Treatment may be entirely inappropriate if the initial problem was not affecting the patient's day-to-day life, especially if intervention could result in the patient having a worse quality of life. Make sure you know the patient's expectations. Why they sought help for the problem and what sort of management they want.

What is the current differential diagnosis?

Why has the patient come to see the doctor?

Was the patient completely well before the onset of this illness?

Box 4.2 SOCRATES: the features of the history of the presenting complaint

- Site
- Onset
- Character
- Radiation
- Associated features
- Timing
- Exacerbating or alleviating features
- Severity

Past medical history

Why ask about past problems, illnesses and surgery? The 'past medical history' (PMH) of a patient is incredibly important for ascertaining whether the patient is generally 'fit and well'. You may discover that the current problems are attributable to a pre-diagnosed condition: certain diagnoses may be excluded if surgery has previously removed the organ under question or the PMH may dictate further management. Certain conditions are often not volunteered or remembered when you ask about the PMH (*see* Box 4.3); for example, high blood pressure (hypertension), ischaemic heart disease (heart attacks, angina), high cholesterol (hypercholesterolaemia), diabetes, epilepsy, asthma or other chest/lung/breathing problems, cancer, rheumatic fever and tuberculosis. Ask about these conditions specifically. Various questions may be required to obtain this information.

> What information might I need to distinguish between the differential diagnoses?

- ➡ 'Have you had any major illnesses in the past?'
- ➡ 'Is there anything you regularly go to your GP for?'
- ➡ 'Have you ever been into hospital before?'
- ➡ 'Are you on any medication for X?'

Box 4.3 Aide-memoire for conditions that may be relevant in a past medical history

- Asthma, anaesthetics
- Blood pressure
- CVA (stroke), cancer
- Diabetes
- Epilepsy
- Fever (rheumatic)
- Gastrointestinal (jaundice)
- High cholesterol
- Infections (TB), ischaemic heart disease (heart attack, angina)

Paediatric history

When taking the history of a child, it is usual to ask questions about the presence of any problems during pregnancy and birth, and about the progression of development. Learn the important developmental milestones of young children. Recall of developmental milestones is easier if you remember the four groups: fine motor and vision; gross motor; hearing and speech; and social. For older children, ask screening questions:

- ➡ 'Does X require additional help at school?'
- ➡ 'Is X at a normal school?'
- ➡ 'Can X keep up with the other students physically and mentally?'

Immunisation history (or lack of it), growth and nutrition are all important in a paediatric history (if not immunised write down the reasons). Information such as this can be found in the child's 'red book', the personal child health record.

Obstetric history

If you are taking the history of a pregnant woman, ask about previous pregnancies, completed and not. Sensitively enquire about abortions (spontaneous and medical), complications with pregnancies and mechanisms of delivery.

Drug history

The patient's 'drug history' (DH) includes past and present medications, recreational drugs and adverse effects of medications. Past medications may have caused an allergic reaction or were ineffective. Either way, you need to make sure the patient is not put back on that medication. If past medications have been effective it is useful to know so they can be tried again. Asking what medications a patient is on often highlights diseases or problems the patient has that they have previously forgotten.

Make a list of the medications the patient is on and ask how long they have been on each one (is this the cause of the presenting complaint?). Does the patient perceive the medication to be effective? For example, how many angina attacks has the patient had since starting long-acting nitrates compared to before?

Over-the-counter, herbal and alternative remedies are important as some interact with commonly used medications. For example, St John's wort (used for depression) can render the oral contraceptive pill less effective.

It can be awkward to ask about recreational drug use. However, it can be important for diagnosis and when identifying social problems. Try; 'I do not want to cause any offence, but I have to ask, do you take . . .' If you get a positive answer about recreational drug use, enquire further about the route (e.g. orally, smoked, injected), quantity and frequency.

Ask specifically about any drug allergies the patient has. Find out the substance and what happened. Specifically, did the patient suffer an anaphylactic reaction?

Family history

Some diseases have a genetic basis. Obtaining an accurate 'family history' (FH) can be useful, not only to manage the patient but also for future management, screening of siblings and children, or both. Illustrate the FH by drawing a family tree. This may clearly reveal a genetic inheritance pattern and enables quick reference. If other members of the family have the same condition as your patient it can be helpful to find out what treatment works for them, as this may also work for your patient.

Social history

The 'social history' (SH) provides information on possible causes of problems (e.g. smoking, alcohol use and occupation). It also directs the management of patients. Investigate the patient's baseline functioning, for example could they dress themselves and climb stairs before coming into hospital? Such information is incredibly useful for discharge planning.

Remember to ask about psychological and social effects of the patient's problems. Certain conditions have strong relationships to depression; however, limitation of lifestyle (work or social) may result in some more subtle negative effects on mood. Ask the patient about their mood to open up this line of enquiry.

Paediatric history

A child's social history will include the ease with which they make friends, favourite lesson, pets and who looks after them. Also ask if they are generally happy. This provides you with further information on development and causes of their presenting complaint and care situation. Details of the parents' or carers' smoking and alcohol habits, occupation, health and relationships is useful, although sensitivity is required so you do not appear to be blaming the parents or carers for the medical condition of the child.

Systems review

Once you have finished your general history it is always a good idea to perform, what is referred to as, a 'systems review' (SR). Ask screening questions, aimed at detecting problems in any system of the body (*see* Table 4.1). These questions will also help you to further investigate the presenting complaint.

TABLE 4.1 Suggestions for questioning during systems review

System	Feature/symptoms to ask about
Cardiovascular system (CVS)	Chest pain, palpitations, sweating, dizziness, limb pain (at rest, on walking), shortness of breath (when, relieving factors), cyanosis, exercise tolerance (what stops the patient first: breathing, leg pain, chest pain?)
Respiratory system (RS)	Chest pain, wheeze, cough, sputum, hoarseness, shortness of breath (when, relieving factors), cyanosis, exercise tolerance
Gastrointestinal system (GI)	Nausea, vomiting, appetite, difficulties swallowing (liquid, solid?), weight loss (intentional?), diarrhoea (mucous, blood?), constipation, steatorrhoea (fatty stools that do not flush away?), change in bowel habit, ulcers (mouth, stomach, intestine?), jaundice
Nervous system (NS)	Headaches, faints, fits, loss of function, loss of sensation, weakness, strokes
Musculoskeletal system (MSS)	Weakness, pain, stiffness (when, duration?), fractures, ability to dress self completely, ability to walk up and down stairs
Genitourinary system (GUS)	Incontinence, frequency, urgency, discharge (urethral, vaginal?), menstruation (last menstrual period, age of first period, regularity, quantity of blood lost, pain?), sexual partners (gender, number, protection used?), pain during sexual intercourse, vaginal bleeding (between periods, after intercourse, after menopause?), hormone therapy (contraceptive or hormone replacement therapy?)

Finishing off

No patient–doctor consultation finishes at the end of the history: a management plan is then developed. As a medical student you may not have the knowledge, or the authority, to construct a management plan; however, you can still practise this final part of the 'history'.

Summarise the patient's main problems. Ask the patient what they want out of their visit and which problems are most important. Tell the patient what will happen next, for example 'I will get the doctor to come and talk to you now' or 'You will probably need a blood test but I will check first'. Check that the patient understands and agrees the management plan before seeking senior help.

As a medical student, you may be taking histories for your own practice. If this is the case make sure you thank the patient. Ask if there is anything they need or want to ask about, so you can discuss this with the consultant team when you present the patient. The patient then also gains benefit through this channel of communication.

Follow up the patients from whom you have taken histories. This will be educationally useful for you, to see what happened next, and also shows the patient respect: that you have not just used them for your needs and then forgotten about them.

MAKING NOTES

Before you make written notes of a patient's history, ask for their consent and ensure confidentiality. If you are writing notes for their clinical file then tell them this. If your notes are for educational purposes, or for discussion with a tutor, you do not need the patient's name or address, so tell the patient this.

Do not write anything during the patient's opening statement. Listen closely to what their presenting complaint is and do not distract them or yourself by writing.

Write only brief notes while you are with the patient. Use prompts for information you feel you would be likely to forget. Write up the notes in full away from the patient. When writing up the notes, make sure you order the history using the template given above, not in the order in which the patient gives you the information. (*See* Chapter 15 for more advice on writing clinical notes.)

TIPS TO HELP YOU PERFECT YOUR HISTORY-TAKING SKILLS

➡ Recap all information obtained at regular intervals and clarify information you are not sure about.
➡ Do not make the patient give information in the order of the template. Structuring the history can help, but rigidity is off-putting and will cause you to lose rapport with the patient and miss information.

➥ When investigating the presenting complaint(s), direct the questions appropriately, rather than just reeling off all the related questions, for example do not ask an 80-year-old lady when her last menstrual period was. An adequate knowledge base assists this.

➥ Do not speak too soon. Allow the patients to talk freely and they will tell you a lot of the information you need to know without the need for prompting.

➥ Present your history to a doctor. There is absolutely no point going through the history-taking process if you receive no feedback. You may be consistently getting something wrong, missing something or going over the top with the information you are obtaining.

➥ Read a clinical skills book to learn more about history-taking and then PRACTISE!

FURTHER READING

Shah N. Taking a history: conclusion and closure. *StudentBMJ*. 2005; **13**: 358–9.
Stride P, Scally P. Better ways of learning. *StudentBMJ*. 2005; **13**: 360–1.

CHAPTER 5

Examination of patients

Physical examination is so important to the General Medical Council (GMC) that it is listed as one of the two fundamental skills required to practise clinical medicine.[1] Good physical examination can accurately determine how 'sick' a patient is. Just by looking at some patients, you can 'spot diagnose' a condition. Read on for the templates for general examination.

Before you can investigate a patient's condition it is essential that you have taken a full history (*see* Chapter 4) and appropriately examined the patient. Examination provides useful information on what is (and is not) abnormal.

Medical school graduates are expected to be proficient in safe and effective examination of a patient's physical and mental state.[2] You are expected to perform intimate examinations of patients of both genders.

Every doctor will tell you a different 'preferred' examination technique. What follows is a general overview of non-emergency patient examination. Read about the full examination of each system in a dedicated clinical examinations book. The examination sequence in an emergency situation, or in a patient you believe is deteriorating, is different and is introduced in Chapter 13.

Follow the rules and advice of those teaching you. In general, as long as you are systematic, confident, safe and caring during the examination you will do well.

RAPPORT

Rapport is essential for full and comfortable physical examination. Patients will have more confidence in you, you become less flustered and the whole experience is less embarrassing for you both.

PERMISSION

Before you examine anyone or anything at anytime, first ask permission. This includes those patients who you want to examine in theatre; gain permission while the patient is still on the ward. Without express permission to examine a patient you can be found guilty of assault or battery. Permission must be given only after a full explanation of what you are going to do, how you are going to do it and why you are doing it (*see* Chapter 2 for information on consent).

Think carefully about how to explain what you are going to do in an examination. Saying 'Is it OK for me to do some tests on your face?' does not sound as appealing as 'Is it OK for me to test the nerves of your head and neck?' when seeking consent to do a cranial nerve examination.

Always remember, patients have a legal right to refuse an examination by a doctor or a medical student. Do not proceed with the examination if your patient is expressing wishes against it.

CHAPERONES

Be aware of what a chaperone is and when one is required. The GMC guidance, *Intimate Examinations*,[3] will guide you in the legal and ethical requirements of performing examinations on the breasts, genitalia or rectum of patients. However, you would be wise to use and offer a chaperone every time you examine a patient.

In addition to national guidance on the use of a chaperone, each health trust and medical school has its own guidance concerning examinations and chaperones. Before you examine patients find out if such publications exist and follow the appropriate advice, guidance and rules.

Examination of children is slightly complicated. Consent from the child can be obtained if they are deemed competent; usually if they are aged 16–17 or are under 16 but 'Gillick competent'. If the child is not competent, seek consent to examine them from the individual with parental responsibility. Do not perform vaginal or rectal examinations on a child (under 18 years) as a medical student and do not examine any child under 16 years old, or under 18 years if incompetent, without a chaperone.

What is a chaperone?

A chaperone is an individual, in addition to the healthcare professional or medical student, who is present to provide patient comfort and support if they are facing an uncomfortable and/or embarrassing examination. Chaperones must have nothing to gain from misinterpreting the events occurring in an examination.[4] Chaperones can have other roles, such as:

➥ assisting with the procedure
➥ undressing the patient if required
➥ interpretation
➥ protection (*see below*).

Chaperones should be the same sex as the patient. Legally and ethically, chaperones are not required to be trained; thus you, as a medical student, can act as a chaperone if the patient is agreeable to this. Relatives or friends of the patient may also be present if the patient so wishes; however, such individuals may coerce with a patient should a complaint be made. Thus, a medical student or healthcare professional chaperone should be offered even if a friend or relative is present as well.

Protection

Unfortunately society is becoming more litigious. Therefore, in addition to providing support and comfort for the patients, chaperones play a role in the protection of both patients and doctors from potentially serious and rare eventualities. A few doctors do pose a danger to patients' safety. To some extent, chaperones can protect the patient's safety by ensuring nothing immoral, unusual, unprofessional or inappropriate occurs during an examination. Similarly, a minority of patients make false or unfair claims of assault against doctors. Use of a chaperone can thus help to prevent such claims being made or assist in the defence of an innocent doctor or medical student. A final, protective role of a chaperone can be to protect the clinician against an attack, although this role is rarely required.

Chaperones cannot provide protection if they are standing behind a door or curtain.[5]

How to use and be a chaperone

If you are performing an intimate examination you must offer a chaperone. Patients can refuse (any chaperone or a particular one) and this must be respected. However, you have no option about whether you should ask. Offer a chaperone for any examination or procedure you are going to perform, intimate or not. As a medical student you should also seek permission from a qualified doctor or nurse to approach the patient and perform the examination. If a chaperone is requested but one is not available, do not carry out the examination.

Chaperones do not guarantee protection of patients or the doctor. Problems can still arise when a chaperone is present, as a result of a questionable need for an intimate examination and poor doctor–patient communication. Therefore, even if you are using a chaperone, make sure the examination is necessary and explain to the patient exactly what you are doing and why you are doing it at each stage of the consent and examination processes. In addition, inappropriate or personal comments to the patient while conducting an examination must not occur. Keep conversation on a topic relevant to what you are doing. If the patient makes an inappropriate comment, or suggests that they are unhappy with the examination, stop immediately.

If a chaperone is present during the examination, record this (and their identity) in the notes. If the patient refuses a chaperone this, too, should be noted.

When you are the chaperone, you must not only establish that the patient is agreeable to having a chaperone but also gain consent for your presence as a medical student.

As a medical student, if you are examining with a chaperone or being the chaperone you can use the experience as a teaching/learning experience. It is recommended that you use senior, qualified health professionals and nurses to act as chaperones, especially when performing intimate examinations.

DIGNITY

When you need to remove items of clothing to perform a thorough examination, only expose the parts required. However, do not be shy: expose enough to allow a thorough examination. You will miss signs if you try and listen to a person's heart through their coat. Use a modesty blanket to cover parts that do not need immediate exposure. Allow the patient to undress and dress in privacy; patients and professionals often find the dressing or undressing stage more embarrassing than a semi-naked examination.

> Do I want a chaperone?

USE YOUR SENSES

Only start your examination once permission has been given and a chaperone is present (when required). Medicine is steeped in tradition and one such tradition is that you approach the patient from their right side to examine them. Practise your examination sequences from the right and it will soon become a habit.

In most cases you will follow the examination sequence of inspection (looking at the patient), palpation (feeling the patient/part of the patient), percussion (*see* Box 5.1) and auscultation (listening, specifically with a stethoscope). This is the traditional examination sequence and is described in every examination book. Although this chapter leads you through the examination in the traditional format it also places emphasis on making full use of all your senses; something neglected by many. Some doctors will tell you that you should use *all* five senses when examining patients; this is mainly good advice, however, some may prefer taste to be an exception.

Sight (inspection)

Use your eyes. You will pick up many diagnoses and a vast amount of information by just looking at the patient and their surroundings. Some disorders can be made from one look alone; a 'spot diagnosis'. Clues from sight can be gained before either you or the patient has said a word. Watch the patient walking into the room, sitting up in bed or using mobility aids. If you are examining a child, watch them play and you will get accurate information on their development.

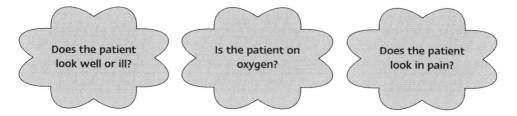

Does the patient look well or ill?

Is the patient on oxygen?

Does the patient look in pain?

Box 5.1 Percussion, the hows and whys

What is percussion?

- A component of a clinical examination that is performed by tapping part of the patient's body with your fingers and interpreting the resulting vibrations. Place your non-dominant hand on the patient's body (often the chest or abdomen) and tap the middle finger with the middle finger of your dominant hand. An exception is percussion of the collarbones (clavicles), for which you tap the bone directly. The best results can be gained by aligning the fingers of the non-dominant hand perpendicular to the direction you will be moving your hand.

Practising percussion

- You must practise. Aim to achieve a loud, clear sound. The tapping should come from the wrist rather than the arm. Percuss anything you can lay your hands on: tables, boxes and your friends. Learn to interpret the different sounds that result.

The information percussion can provide

- Percussion allows you to determine if fluid, tissue or air underlies the surface you are percussing. Normally, the chest and abdomen will sound resonant. The sound is dull if there is fluid or tissue present underneath; this is heard normally, for example, over the liver. If excess air is present the percussion 'note' becomes 'hyper-resonant'. You will have to practise to understand the difference between these. The uses of percussion are thus to detect the abnormal presence of fluid (e.g. free within the abdomen (ascites) or around the lungs (pleural effusion)), tissue (e.g. enlarged organs) or excess air (e.g. emphysema, air around the lung (pneumothorax)).

Be systematic at all times, even when examining the patient visually. Look around the surroundings for medical instruments, vomit or sputum and the positioning of the patient (bed, chair, wheelchair?). Unfortunately, (and perhaps cynically) you may also spot signs of bad habits; for example, biscuits or sweets next to a diabetic whose blood sugar is out of control, or crisps and fizzy drinks in the bag of an outpatient who says he or she cannot

What clues to diagnosis lie around the patient?

understand why they have put on three stone in one year when they cannot eat anything. Assess the patient directly for comfort, their colour (blue (cyanosed), yellow (jaundiced)); is the patient flushed, are there any scars, injuries (including piercings and tattoos), bruising; observe nutrition, ease of breathing and respiratory rate and mobility.

Some screening tests may be appropriate before you look at the patient more closely. For example, ask a patient complaining of a sore shoulder to put their hands behind their head, behind their lower back and reach one hand over the opposite shoulder. If a patient can perform all of these manoeuvres the chance of them having significant pathology in the shoulder is much reduced. Similarly, you may ask a patient to walk at the beginning of your examination to assess for a limp or muscle weakness. Positive findings at this stage allow you to quickly refine your examination.

Next, approach the patient for closer examination. Start at the hands; look at the skin, joints, nails and movement. Disgusting it may be, but information can even be gained from finding excrement in a patient's finger nails; something often accompanying dementia (the clinical examination books never seem to mention this).

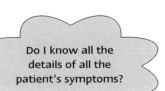

What are the causes of finger clubbing?

Incorporate touch to feel the radial pulse (this looks neater than going back to it when you get to the 'touch' part of the examination) and blood pressure. Go on up to the eyes and examine for jaundice, fatty deposits and anaemia, then move down to the mouth and tongue. Then finally look at the chest wall, abdomen or other focus of the examination. Re-examine these parts more closely, looking again for scars (some hide in unusual places), lumps, bumps or growths, abnormal movements and system specific signs.

Do I know all the details of all the patient's symptoms?

Taste

Many experienced doctors have been known to say the five senses are all used in gaining information on a patient. Yet it is extremely unusual to see any of the aforementioned professionals use taste in a diagnosis. The classic scenario is a doctor tasting a patient's urine for sugar; they will always tell you that is what used to happen in the 'good old days'. However, in reality the closest you will ever get to using taste is assessing the patient's choice of confectionery while sampling their sweets when offered. Harmless as this may sound, caution must be exercised even for this, raisins rarely come loose in a bowl of sweets . . . perhaps they used to be covered in chocolate!

Smell

Various infections (*Clostridium difficile*, candida), high levels of ketones, and constipated patients, among a plethora of conditions, have a distinctive smell to the experienced nose.

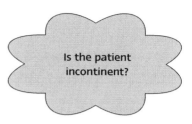

Is the patient incontinent?

Touch (palpation and percussion)

DO NOT touch a patient until you are sure you have gained as much information on a patient from the other two (or three) senses as you possibly can. Touch can provide a massive array of information on a patient's condition: identification of lumps and bumps, temperature, texture and a previously unknown source of pain.

Ask the patient if they have any pain anywhere before you touch them; rapport and respect are quickly lost (and exams can be failed) if you hurt your patient. If the patient states that they have pain, start your examination as far away from this pain as you can, leave the tender part until last. Similarly, if the patient has two of the body part you are examining (e.g. most patients have two hands, two legs, etc.), examine the normal side first; this gives you a normal 'baseline' to compare with the troublesome side.

Touch the patient only lightly to begin with. Gain information on temperature, texture, tenderness and anatomy, as appropriate. If light touch elicits pain do not progress to more firm or deep palpation in the affected area. While palpating a patient, always watch their face for signs of pain, discomfort or distress.

During abdominal examination, how do you distinguish between the spleen and a kidney?

Another form of touch involves percussion (*see* Box 5.1 above). This technique provides information on how dense the underlying tissues are and can help you to identify the normal or abnormal presence of organs, air or fluid.

Sound (auscultation)

'Oh, now I can hear it!' I would say, my ears strained to the stethoscope. But above the hum of the daily activity of the hospital I couldn't hear the heartbeat at all, let alone a super-added murmur caused by turbulent flow through a dodgy valve. Baffling! Years later, in the calm and hush or my own practice, all became clear and I started hearing things that I didn't even know existed.[6]

The wheezing of an asthmatic, the clickety-click of mechanical heart valves and the whining of malingering patients (who said that?) provide great information on past medical history, current condition and patients' airways. Such information can be gained while generally assessing the patient and throughout the examination.

A more specific use of sound is implemented at the end of the examination sequence: auscultation. Appropriate body parts are 'listened to' with a stethoscope. You may listen for heart sounds, murmurs (turbulent blood flow through heart valves), disorders of the lung (bronchial breathing, crackles), bowel sounds or bruits (turbulent flow through blood vessels).

Special tests

Nearly all body systems have their own special tests or further investigations that are so crucial they become part of the examination. For each examination you perform, learn these 'special tests'. For example, abdominal examination should include examination for hernias, examination of external genitalia and rectal examination ('if you don't put your finger in it, you put your foot in it'). Further, you should also check the patient's urine for blood, sugar or infection.

Examination of a child must include reference to the child's 'red book', the personal child health record. The red book, usually issued by a health visitor, is carried by the mother and contains details of the child's birth, growth, weight, development, immunisations and check-ups. Much can be gained from the red book so familiarise yourself with its contents early in a paediatric placement.

Common sense

Common sense is crucial.
➥ Do not ask the patient to do something they are incapable of doing.
➥ Do not hurt the patient.
➥ Only examine what you have been asked to/what is required.
➥ Finally, do not follow rigid templates when examining children. Take advantage of situations when the child is quiet to listen to the heart and lungs, and do not insist on the child being on a couch for examination.

SYSTEM TEMPLATES

To recapitulate, the general template for examining bodily systems is organised into inspection, palpation, percussion and auscultation. Knowing any specific signs for each system works well for examination of the following systems.
➥ Cardiovascular (heart and blood vessels)
➥ Gastrointestinal (mouth to anus, liver and pancreas)
➥ Genitourinary (waterworks and genitals)
➥ Respiratory (airways).

The template can be adapted for obstetric (pregnant women) examination. However, musculoskeletal (muscles, bones and joints) and neurological (brain and nerves) examinations require different templates.

Musculoskeletal template

The musculoskeletal template consists of *look*, *feel* and *move*.

➡ Look for redness, swelling, deformity and scars.

➡ Feel for temperature, tenderness and swellings.

➡ Move the joints. Examine active (the patient does it independently) and passive movements (you are moving the body part for the patient).

Examine the joint(s) in question and the ones just above and below.

> What tests can you perform to examine the stability of the knee?

> What are the different features of upper and lower motor neurone lesions?

For example, a knee examination also includes the hip and ankle. Assess the blood and nerve supply to the surrounding body parts and the function of the joint being examined; can the patient perform their normal activities of daily living? For example, can the patient do the following.

➡ Do up buttons? (hands)

➡ Comb their hair? (shoulder)

➡ Manage stairs? (knee)

➡ Get in and out of a car? (hip)

➡ Tie their shoelaces? (back).

Neurological template

The neurological template is the most different from all the others. After assessing cognitive function (thought processes) and cranial nerves (nerves supplying the head and neck), the remaining neurological examination is ordered into *appearance*, *tone* (how floppy or stiff the limb is), *power* (how strong the limb is), *reflexes*, *co-ordination* and *sensation*. You will need to know how to test each of these specifically for the upper and lower limbs, and be able to determine between upper and lower motor neurone signs.

SAY WHAT YOU SEE

As a medical student you will often have to report your findings, verbally or in the patient's notes. Be structured, organised and concise (just like your examination). State the positive and any relevant negative findings. Do not state all the negatives, especially in the exam situation this will only serve as a source of awkward questioning.

> Am I able to examine all 12 cranial nerves in sequence without forgetting any?

During your career you will be examining patients in order to help you come to a conclusion on their diagnosis. Remember this when examining a patient as a medical student. Do not say you can feel, see or hear what the student before you has said, and do not say you can feel something you cannot just because you think that is what your tutor wants you to say. Report your findings accurately and honestly. The person before you may have been mistaken or you may need further guidance on how to find a specific sign.

FINAL WORDS

When you are learning examinations, ensure that the general approach is at the forefront of your mind; it does not matter if you cannot remember each part of examination in detail if you know to inspect, palpate, percuss and auscultate. It can be useful to write down examination sequences (including any screening and special tests and investigations). This will encourage you to run through your examinations in your mind, on non-medical family or friends or on your teddy bear!; having it in written form prevents you from forgetting the same thing on each examination and ensures you know the routine inside out.

Practise on everybody you can. Only with repeated exposure to normal findings will abnormal findings become more obvious. You will gain information efficiently if you are structured, systematic and slick. This will build the patient's confidence in you and will help your own confidence. Try and experience as many abnormal signs as you can. You need to learn what an enlarged liver feels like, how to elicit shifting dullness and how to define a heart murmur before you are left to do such things independently.

> To assist your interpretation of findings, practise examination alongside a skeleton or anatomy book. Learn the anatomical structures that lie beneath your hands (and eyes) during each part of the examination.

FURTHER READING

Brain (a neurological journal). *Aids to the Examination of the Peripheral Nervous System*, 4th ed. Edinburgh: WB Saunders; 2004.

Bignell CJ. Chaperones for genital examination provide comfort and support for the patient and protection for the doctor. *BMJ.* 1999; **319**: 137–8.

Kulkarni K. Three's a crowd. *StudentBMJ.* 2005; **13**: 458–60.

Munro JF, Campbell IW. *Macleod's Clinical Examination*, 10th ed. Edinburgh: Churchill Livingstone; 2000.

CHAPTER 6

Presenting patients

A perfect history and a thorough examination are worthless without effective communication of your findings to other healthcare professionals.

No history or examination is complete without presentation of the case. As a junior doctor you will have to 'hand over' or 'present' new patients to your seniors on ward rounds, and you will use the skill to hand over patients you are worried about to on-call doctors. Learn how to communicate your findings in a clear, succinct and ordered manner. As a medical student, presentation to doctors also allows the opportunity for assessment of your history and examination skills. Finally, as a medical school graduate you are required to be able to interpret findings from your history and examination of patients. Presenting a patient's case, management plan and your impression of the likely diagnosis will illustrate your competency in this interpretation.[1]

BASIC FORMAT FOR PRESENTATION OF A PATIENT

The information you present must be clear and accurate for effective patient care and clear understanding. Misrepresentation of information can result in inaccurate diagnoses and unnecessary, missed and/ or dangerous investigation or treatment.

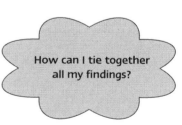

How can I tie together all my findings?

Introduce the patient

Illustrate the patient's 'normal life' by introducing who they are and not just their problems. State the patient's:

➡ name (including preferred name, if different)
➡ age
➡ occupation
➡ relevant social situation, such as lives alone, recently widowed; for example, 'This is John Smith, a 70-year-old retired publican who cares for his wife.'

Brief summary

Provide information on the current health (or not) of the patient by tying in relevant past medical history with the current problem:

➥ give a chronological account of directly related past medical history, for example 'This man is a known arteriopath who had a myocardial infarction (heart attack) one year ago.'

➥ state the recent symptoms, for example 'He has had increasing frequency of chest pain on exertion for the past month.'

➥ describe the current problems, for example 'John presented today with ongoing chest pain for the past hour, radiating down the left arm, associated with shortness of breath, nausea and sweating.'

Relevant past medical history in conventional and chronological order

Expand what you have just said about the patient's past history and current complaint. If you miss something, leave it out unless it is really important (late inclusion causes confusion). When expanding your introduction:

➥ use the patient's words to describe their symptoms.

➥ if you are unsure which illnesses the patient has had, present the term(s) they used.

➥ do not use abbreviations.

➥ include relevant aetiological (causative) or risk factors, for example 'John has smoked 20 cigarettes a day for 35 years (35 pack-year history), he was diagnosed with diabetes 15 years ago and has been treated for high blood pressure for the past 10 years. Last year he had a myocardial infarction and was treated with thrombolysis. He has only had two episodes of angina since.'

From the drug, family and social history, only present relevant information; however, make sure your notes are thorough, for example 'John currently takes aspirin, a simvastatin and ramipril. John's father died aged 45 years of a myocardial infarction. John currently has no significant limitation to his exercise tolerance. He lives in a house with stairs and manages these well.'

Examination findings

Even if you have performed the most thorough examination of your life, only present the positive findings and relevant negative findings. Irrelevant minutiae will waste time. Present the examination in the order in which you carry it out, for example 'On inspection I found . . .', 'On palpation there was . . .', etc.

Summarise your history succinctly

The aim of presenting a history is to let another professional know about the patient's condition. You should state what you are going to say using the introduction mentioned above. Say what you want to say by recounting the pertinent points of the history. Then say what you have said, summarise the case in just a couple of lines incorporating the differential diagnoses you have devised (*see below*).

Give a list of differential diagnoses

Patients may remain undiagnosed at first presentation. Therefore, the most likely or important (e.g. life-threatening) diagnoses are listed and need ruling out first. These diagnoses are the 'differential diagnoses'. If a doctor has already seen the patient, differential diagnoses should be documented. However, these are not gospel and you need practice so try and formulate your own list of differential diagnoses. If the patient has been in hospital, or has been ill for a while, you can present the working diagnosis. However, think of possible alternatives, these will be relevant if current management is not successful. For example, 'This is John Smith, a 70-year-old gentleman who had a myocardial infarction one year ago. He has presented again with cardiac-sounding chest pain and I would like to rule out acute coronary syndrome.'

Test results

Tests should be done only after a full history and examination have taken place. Their main role is to exclude or confirm differential diagnoses.

Be familiar with and present relevant test results, especially those you think require discussion or you are unsure about. If tests have not been done, formulate a list of tests in the order in which you believe they should be done and present these. This is difficult for junior medical students, but it is an important skill to master. Look in textbooks for recommended tests for the given/your differential diagnoses. Remember, start basic, non-invasive and cheap, and work up to the more complicated, invasive and/or expensive tests.

The management plan

Present the management to date and construct a possible future management plan. Patients must always be involved in management planning, therefore speak to the patient about what they want, what they have already been told and what their ultimate goal is.

Placement of the patient

Depending on the state of the patient and their social situation, inpatient management may be most appropriate. What sort of ward would meet their needs (e.g. intensive care, high-dependency, specialised, general)? If outpatient care is appropriate, will the patient need additional support?

Aim of the management

Is cure or symptom control the aim of the management plan? Palliative treatment is aimed at symptom management rather than cure. Consider where the patient wants to die and whether their spiritual concerns are managed.

Urgency of treatment

Does something need doing right now, today, tomorrow, in the next week or month or can it wait for a few years? What can you do now to improve the situation?

Preventative treatment can be undertaken to stop the condition getting any worse, or to stop another condition from occurring. This may include giving up smoking, reducing alcohol intake and taking more exercise.

Further management resources

Are external agencies required in the management of the patient? External agencies have a role in both short and long-term settings, for example social services.

Patients and their family or friends will often have questions and concerns that do not occur to them at the time of diagnosis or management planning. Think about sources of further support and advice should they need any questions answering, for example leaflets, websites, the Patient Advice and Liaison Services (PALS).

Patient Advice and Liaison Services (PALS)

Involve the whole team

Multi-disciplinary team working is crucial to effective patient care. Always consider the multi-disciplinary team and expand on the roles of each member, at all relevant stages of the management plan.

Present at least one patient on each formal ward round that you attend.

FURTHER READING

Beasley R, Bernau S, Aldington S, Robinson G. From medical student to junior doctor: the medical handover – a good habit to cultivate. *StudentBMJ*. 2006; **14**: 188–9.

National Health Service National Patient Safety Agency, National Health Service Modernisation Agency, British Medical Association. *Safe Handover: safe patients – guidance on clinical handover for clinicians and managers*. London: British Medical Association. (Available at: www.saferhealthcare.org.uk/NR/rdonlyres/0F86311C-3B4B-4392-8FF6-4A5B7EE50D2D/0/Safe_Handover_Safe_Patients.pdf)

Patient Advice and Liaison Services (PALS): www.dh.gov.uk/PolicyAnd Guidance/OrganisationPolicy/PatientAndPublicInvolvement/PatientAdvice AndLiaisonServices/fs/en and www.pals.nhs.uk.

CHAPTER 7

Ward life and rounds

Varying in size, time and educational benefit, ward rounds depend largely on the professional leading them, but there is etiquette involved in ward life and rounds. So what is expected of medical students on the wards and during ward rounds?

Medical students are required to learn about surgical and peri-operative care, recognising and managing acute illness, palliative care, and relieving pain and distress.[1] Where better to learn than on the wards?

Medical schools try to place you on wards that are appropriate to the module you are studying; however, owing to numerous medical students and a lack of specialist wards in some hospitals this is not always possible. If you are not placed on a directly module-related ward, do not worry. The vast majority (if not all) of your basic skills can be learnt on any ward.

WARD LIFE
Befriend the ward staff

> The most important thing you have to do on the ward is get on with the nurses
> . . . upset the ward sister and you will never recover.

The nurses and the ward clerk (if present) are the backbone of the ward. They know the patients and the ward inside out: the times of appointments, social situations, who to ring to book an investigation, and so on.

Befriending the ward staff can sometimes be easier said than done. Some ward staff may dislike or be ambivalent towards all medical students. Perhaps those before you have been rude, there may not be enough physical space for you and you are only temporary. This can be hard to overcome. Do not take it personally, just try that little bit harder to show that you are eager to help as well as learn.

Introduce yourself to all ward staff as soon as you get on the ward. All healthcare professionals are busy people, if you do not make an effort nor will they. Catch the members of each team at a good time to introduce yourself and explain what you want to do during your time on the ward.

Although you are training to be a doctor, this does not mean you cannot help the nurses. Offer assistance to the nurses and they will help you out in return. If you are practising how to take blood or are putting in an intravenous cannula, and you spill some blood on the sheet, make sure you change it. If you do not know where the bed linen is kept, or where you should put dirty laundry, then ask. Whatever you do, do not leave a mess.

Healthcare assistants are the members of the nursing staff who have not been to nursing college. They are not 'untrained nurses'. Healthcare assistants look after the basic needs of the patients (e.g. washing, dressing, toileting and feeding) and perform administrative duties on the ward. Healthcare assistants are often valuable sources of useful information, such as how much the patients are eating and drinking and how much and what is coming out of both ends.

Many healthcare assistants and qualified nurses will be the same age as you. You may form good friendships among ward staff that continue after your placement ends.

Do not forget about the domestic assistants on the ward. Crucial members of the ward team, domestic assistants provide patients with those treasured cups of tea and coffee. Domestic assistants are also responsible for cleaning the ward. Without them, many more patients would contract infections. Involve domestics in the ward team. A smile and/or a hello every time you encounter them on the ward will go a long way and will ensure you do not appear arrogant.

Learn the arrangement of the consultant team

During hospital placements, you will usually be placed within a consultant-led team. These teams differ between and within each hospital. Differences between teams arise from workload, consultant or trust preference and available facilities.

Some teams have one consultant and are pyramidal in design. There may be three or four house officers (HOs) or Foundation Year 1 (FY1) doctors, two or three senior house officers (SHOs) or Foundation Year 2 (FY2) doctors, one or two registrars and one consultant. Other teams may be linear, with equal numbers of HOs/FY1s, SHOs/FY1s, registrars and consultants.

Understand the set-up of your team as early as possible, find out:

➡ how many consultants comprise the team
➡ the grades or positions of each team member
➡ the name and pager number for each member
➡ the times of ward rounds (and theatre lists)
➡ which patients you are involved with.

Multi-disciplinary teams

Multi-disciplinary team working is increasingly popular. Often consultant-led, a multi-disciplinary team consists of a number of different types of healthcare professionals: medical and/or surgical doctors, nurses, specialist nurses, physiotherapists, occupational therapists, dieticians, radiologists, social workers and psychologists.

Multi-disciplinary teams were introduced to encourage a streamlined and efficient approach to patient care. Regular multi-disciplinary team meetings ensure efficient communication, discussion of problems and development of thoroughly thought-through management plans. Each multi-disciplinary team member should be aware of the patient-agreed management plan, which results in less confusion for the patients.

Multi-disciplinary teams are good for patient care because they cultivate an environment of sharing knowledge from a wide range of backgrounds. The varied training and experiences result in a different approach to problems by each team member; the patient's problems are dealt with in a more holistic way through thorough discussion.

Unfortunately, multi-disciplinary teams are not without problems. Discussion can result in disagreement. Different healthcare professionals have their own targets, which may not be the same as those of their colleagues. Disagreement can lead to ongoing conflict, which can lead to a breakdown of communication. Inadequate or damaged communication can result in duplicated work, unidentified roles in patient care and gaps in service provision.

As a medical student you can benefit from the advantages and disadvantages of multi-disciplinary teams. Your education will be enriched by the views and problems faced by each healthcare profession. You will gain an understanding of the different roles, which can only be helpful when planning the management of a patient. Analyse why conflict has occurred and think of solutions or prevention strategies to stop finding yourself in the same situation in the future.

Much can be learnt from other healthcare professionals. Ask members of your multi-disciplinary team if you can spend time with them. Follow a patient from presentation, through treatment and rehabilitation, to discharge, if possible follow them up as an outpatient. Social workers and specialist nurses often have vast amounts of knowledge on all aspects of the patient. It can be a mutually beneficial arrangement in terms of sharing medical knowledge. Professionals who spend all of their time in one specialty will be hugely knowledgeable about that area; for example, you may learn more from a specialist nurse than you would from a consultant. However, you may have a more in-depth knowledge of topics unrelated to that specialty. If unrelated issues do arise you may be able to share your knowledge with the individual.

How to work effectively in a team

Whether you are working in a multi-disciplinary team or a group of medical students, you require effective team-working skills. In your postgraduate career, if you are a poor team member you will make your colleagues' life difficult and a misery. Qualities required for successful team working should be held by all and are described below.

➡ *Trust and honesty.* Without these two important qualities you will waste time checking your team-mates' work. If you are not honest, they will be checking up on you.

➡ *Good communication skills.* There is no point doing something if your team-mates do not know you have done it; work will be duplicated. Similarly, you may not know something needs to be done without being told. Goals will be achieved more quickly and effectively, and understanding will be increased if you communicate your work and knowledge.

➡ *Support.* Be there for each other. Emotional and professional support is required throughout your undergraduate and postgraduate training. Make it a two-way process.

➡ *Compromise.* All team members want to further their expertise and skills. Sometimes compromise is required for all to get a fair exposure to new experiences. However, one area in which compromise should not take place is patient care.

➡ *Organisation.* Organisation significantly reduces working time. Know what each other is doing and do your own jobs in a logical, organised way; you will have much more time to spend on each activity. Organise a team leader. Teams run much more smoothly with a designated leader. Distribute work fairly to ensure no one is more overworked than the others.

> Doctors are not intrinsically good team players. We are trained to be competitive and are regarded for surpassing others. Most of us are not taught how to work effectively in teams; it is widely seen as a part of our personality – you are either good at it or not. Once we enter the hospital environment, inevitably we have difficulty working alongside peers or colleagues with varying mental abilities and backgrounds.[2]

➡ *Professionalism.* You may not like all team members but you should respect and behave in a professional manner towards them at all times. Put forward a united front, otherwise all work will be undermined.

➡ *Knowing each members' boundaries.* Know what each team member is capable of and allowed to do. Work around restraints and do not pressure team members to do things they are not comfortable with. If you feel forced to do more than you are allowed to, communicate this. If you are not allowed to do as much as you wish, inform your team members and try to reach a solution.

➡ *Ability to resolve conflict.* At times conflict will arise and each member of the team must work hard to resolve this. Allow each member to state their problems, understand each others' roles and ensure everybody understands the common goals.

If you are working in a team and are finding it difficult, have a look through the above qualities and evaluate each member's accordingly. Can you identify the factor that is letting the team down? How can you address this? Sometimes the answer is to just grin and bear it until your placement ends but practise the skill of improving teamwork while you are a medical student; it is something you will need to do when you are a doctor.

Refining clinical skills

The wards provide opportunity to learn many of the clinical skills required of medical students. At convenient times track down appropriate members of staff to watch and learn from them. When you feel ready, ask to be supervised in performing the skill yourself. Skills involving drugs or prescriptions can be practised with unbelievable frequency. Learn to work out drug dosages, write prescriptions and witness the administration of medications. You may be allowed to administer medication via intramuscular (im; into the muscle), intravenous (iv; into the vein), subcutaneous (sc; into the fat under the skin) injections, nasogastric (NG; tube from nose to stomach) or gastrostomy (tube through abdominal wall into stomach) routes. You may even be able to insert a NG tube. Learn about nebulisers (machines that use compressed gas to vaporise medication for inhalation), how to set them up and the drugs that are given via this route.

Patients often complain about 'feeling like pincushions' or are surprised they 'have any blood left'. This is not just a result of the presence of eager medical students, but the practice of regular blood-sampling in hospital. Get in on the action. You need to be able to take venous and arterial blood, and to insert venous cannulae ('drip needles'). Ask the nurses to let you know when these are required; it may take the job off their hands.

When practising taking blood, the job does not finish as you place the needle in the yellow tub and wash your hands. You must learn how to label the samples and fill out request forms correctly. Once the bloods have been processed you should attempt to interpret the results. Do this regularly and the normal values of the common blood tests will soon be second nature to you. Reflect on how useful each blood test was and whether you would do it again in the same situation in the future. Are any further tests required as a result of the blood tests? Can you explain the results? Do the results fit with the patient's clinical condition? If you are unsure, ask one of the doctors – you may be able to work through these questions together.

Unfortunately, cardiac arrest and collapse are not uncommon on hospital wards. Take advantage of these events by gaining exposure, experience and practice of cardiopulmonary resuscitation and advanced life-support while you are still in the comfort zone of being a student. Associated with this (and the daily ward routine) is the administration of oxygen therapy. Learn how to work oxygen administration equipment, understand how much oxygen should be given in various situations and when oxygen should be used with care.

The labour ward can be a great experience, but is also very frustrating at times. You can spend over 10 hours with a patient in labour, hoping to deliver her baby, only for her to have a Caesarean section at the last minute.

You must understand that it is inappropriate for you to walk into the room of a woman in labour at the last minute and expect to deliver the baby. Instead, you should spend time with the mother throughout the labour, helping out and encouraging her. Become a familiar and friendly face and you will be seen as being helpful, rather than simply standing and watching her in a lot of pain! Attend the labour ward with the intention of following only a couple of ladies per shift, and you may see them deliver their babies.

Arrive at the labour ward before the midwife co-ordinator 'hands-over' patients from the previous shift – this may mean going in very early. This is one of the first steps in earning respect from the midwives – you have shown that you are willing to get up as early as they do. The 'hand-over' is also a good time to be placed with a midwife for the day, thus informing you of which patients you will be involved with.

Be as helpful as possible. Find out where blankets, equipment, gloves, etc., are kept so that you can get them quickly when necessary. Offer to monitor your patient's blood pressure, pulse and temperature regularly for the midwife; this is another way of getting to know the patient. If a patient is sick, don't just stand there and watch, put on some gloves and wipe it up. The patient and the midwife will really appreciate these simple things.

The next important thing to talk about is tea and coffee. Midwives drink a lot of tea and coffee, and they will usually be happy for you to join them. However, *the staff members often pay for the drinks* so make sure that you contribute to the fund during your placement. If you are at a loose end offer to make the midwives a drink. After a lady has given birth she is usually offered something to eat and drink. It is usually the healthcare assistants who do this; if they are not available, take the initiative and do it yourself.

You do not have to stay for a full shift. Definitely stay if you are getting good experience and are being useful and helpful. If there is not much to do and the end of the shift is nearing, ask whether there is anything else you can help with. If there is nothing to do, the midwives usually do not mind if you ask if you can leave.

Last of all, if you feel that you have had a good experience on the labour ward after a placement, and you have got on well with the staff, bake them a cake or buy some biscuits to take in on your last day to say 'thank you'. You need not spend a lot, but it is really appreciated. *(Ali Williams, fourth-year medical student, Leeds)*

Bladder catheterisation involves inserting a tube via the urethra (connects the bladder with the external genitalia) into the bladder to drain urine. Doctors are often only asked to perform this on males; however, you should practise inserting urinary catheters into males and females. This skill requires a chaperone and fully informed consent owing to its intimate nature. Other opportunities to do this will commonly arise in the operating theatre; however, you *must* ask the patient's consent before they are anaesthetised in order to perform this procedure.

> Does the patient have a previous similar X-ray with which I can compare the most recent one?

Medical students are commonly asked to interpret chest and abdominal radiographs (X-rays); common investigations from which a lot of information may be gained. Only by looking at vast numbers of radiographs will you be able to identify abnormal appearances quickly. Make sure you know whether a radiograph is normal, and if not, whether the abnormality is clinically relevant, indicates a diagnosis or indicates the need for further investigation.[3] For thorough interpretation of radiographs you need to learn a sequence such as the following.

➡ Check the name, date of birth and sex of the patient.
➡ Determine the date of the radiograph.
➡ What the radiograph is an image of.
➡ Identify the orientation, projection (whether it was taken from front to back, back to front or from the side), whether the patient was standing or lying, the exposure (how well the tissues of interest can be visualised) and rotation (if the patient is viewed straight on or at an angle)
➡ Are there any glaring abnormalities?
➡ Look at specific features; for example, **a**lignment, **b**ones, **c**artilage and **s**oft tissues/organs (ABCS).
➡ Are there additional, abnormal or foreign features? For example, air or fluid where it should not be, abnormal calcification, stones (gallstones or kidney stones) and iatrogenic factors (resulting from activities of health professionals) such as mechanical heart valves, wires or clips, coils and pacemakers. Be alert to buttons, cardiac monitor pads, coils, piercings and bra underwires; do not assume all abnormal features of a radiograph are within the body.

Devise a sequence that is logical to you. If you have access to the patients' previous radiographs view them with the current one to detect subtle changes. While you are learning always try and interpret the radiograph before looking at any reports. If a report does not agree with your interpretation try and make sense of the differences and identify the abnormalities described in the report.

A similar system can be used for the interpretation of computed tomography (CT) scans and magnetic resonance imaging (MRI) scans. Remember to interpret these scans as if you are looking at the slices of the body from the patient's feet looking up as they are lying on their back. Identify major anatomical features and look for symmetry; asymmetry may alert you to a problem. Understand the basics of how the images are obtained, which imaging technique is preferable for the major structures of the body and how images may be enhanced with contrast or changing the settings to improve interpretation. Try to go along with some of your patients to the scanning rooms, with the radiographer's permission. You will see what having each scan involves and, if the radiographer is in a good mood and is not too busy, you may get a short tutorial from the experts on interpretation.

WARD ROUNDS

In general, medical ward rounds take longer than surgical ones; medical teams can spend half a day seeing their patients. Surgical ward rounds usually start early, often at 8 am so the patients can be quickly seen before the theatre list starts at 9 am.

➡ *Carry your stethoscope.* Make sure you do not miss any interesting signs as a result of not having your stethoscope. In addition, senior doctors do not always carry their stethoscope and medical students are often promoted to 'chief stethoscope lenders'.

➡ *Arrive in good time.* Try to arrive 15 minutes before the ward round. This has many advantages: you have time to be late, the consultant may turn up early and you can gather or help to gather the last-minute investigation results.

➡ *Take a pen and paper with you.* You never know when you will be told a pearl of knowledge that you want to note down. Pens also come in handy if you are asked to record details in the patient's notes (and you may also get promoted to 'chief pen lender' as well as your seniors will not always have these either).

➡ *Know the patients.* Nothing will upset your consultant more than you not knowing the patients. Clerk (take a history and examine) as many patients as you can. At the very least, familiarise yourself with patients' cases by reading their notes. Look up relevant test results. Be familiar with all the available radiographs so you could easily present them if asked. Devise a differential diagnosis and management plan; if these are wrong you may feel a little silly, but if you are right it will boost your confidence and put a large smile on your consultant's face.

➡ *Ensure the nursing staff are aware the ward round is about to start so they can join in.* Nursing staff often know the most about the patients' progress and the presence of a nurse on the ward round encourages good inter-professional communication, thus improving patient management.

➡ *Ensure patient dignity.* Help make sure curtains are closed (and opened at the end of visit).

➥ *Help patients to sit up.* Often a patient's chest will need examining and they cannot sit forwards to have their back auscultated. Use your presence constructively by assisting the patient to sit forwards.

➥ *Clean your hands between each and every patient.* Methycillin or multi-resistant *Staphylococcus aureus* (MRSA), *Clostridium difficile* (*C. diff*) . . . need more be said?

➥ *Help to locate clinical notes before the ward round starts.* It becomes stressful for everyone if the consultant starts getting agitated and irritable because the notes for the next patient are missing.

➥ *Help the junior doctors.* Practise writing in the medical notes (write what you think is correct then get another doctor to check and countersign what you have written), fetch paper or investigation request forms (you will learn the layout of the ward and what things look like) and write down jobs that the consultant is giving the team to do to help ensure nothing is missed.

➥ *Ensure you have had a good breakfast or lunch.* Eating well before the ward round will enable your energy level to remain adequate throughout.

➥ *Know where the toilets are along the route of the ward round.* If you receive a call of nature you may have difficulty postponing it until the end of a long ward round. Try to slip to the toilet between wards or bays. No decent doctor would be able to refuse you, just don't make a habit of it!

➥ *Be on the ball.* You need to think and move quickly, know who and what is coming next and be prepared for it.

➥ *Respond to questions promptly.* If a consultant fires a question at you have confidence in yourself to provide an answer. It does not matter if you answer a question incorrectly: the humiliation ensures you will never forget that answer. If you do not know the answer say so, stalling will not make the question disappear and will waste everybody's time.

FURTHER READING

Corne J, Carroll M, Brown I *et al. Chest X-ray Made Easy*, 2nd ed. Edinburgh: Churchill Livingstone; 2002.

Dosani S. Getting the most out of your house officer. *StudentBMJ.* 2001; **9**: 117.

Harris R, Fitzgerald I. Tips on getting teaching on the wards. *StudentBMJ.* 2005; **13**: 333.

King J. Tackling troubled teams. *BMJ Career Focus.* 2005; **331**: 115–16.

CHAPTER 8

Clinics

Clinics can be really useful; however, some can be a total waste of time. Learn to judge the value of a clinic during your clinical years and only attend those that will be of use (or are compulsory).

Clinics are usually for outpatients who have a medical condition that does not require inpatient treatment but needs expert evaluation or monitoring. However, inpatients may attend clinics for problems aside from those that have led to their current admission. Clinics may be held in an outpatient department, offices within a main hospital or a GP surgery or health centre.

Clinics are attended by consultants (or a member of their team), GPs or both. Increasingly, specialist nurses run their own clinics. However, other healthcare professionals may also be available to see patients in clinic, and they can be a rich source of knowledge and education, for example dieticians, psychologists and technicians.

You may be expected to attend clinics as part of your placement timetable. However, if there are particular clinics that you think will be useful you can ask permission to attend by ringing the secretary or professional directly to arrange a time and date.

WHAT CLINICS DO FOR YOU

Your seniority as a medical student, and the professional holding the clinic, will dictate what you will be allowed to do. However, being aware of what may be available will allow you to suggest activities you would like to undertake.

Junior medical students may sit in with one of the healthcare professionals and observe clinic appointments. Although non-interactive clinic experiences carry the least educational benefit, they can be a good introduction if you are scared, inexperienced or both. The professional you are with may ask you questions, or ask you to ask the patient further questions. This will gently ease you into the next step . . . seeing patients on your own.

Take any available opportunities to see patients on your own. This is sometimes not possible because of lack of space, which may be inadequate for you to have your own private room. However, seeing new patients on your own can be a valuable lesson in concise history and examination skills.

Less frequently you may be asked to see, or be involved in seeing, old patients returning for a follow-up appointment after tests or investigations. This will enable you to practise your interpretation and management planning skills in the safety of the clinic environment where emergency medicine is not usually a feature.

Clinics provide the opportunities to learn or practise general (e.g. general examination, communication) and specialty-specific skills. The latter may include respiratory function tests, digital rectal examination or proctoscopy (using a short instrument to visualise the rectum) and foetal heartbeat monitoring.

TIPS FOR GETTING ALONG WELL IN CLINIC

➡ *Identify the clinic co-ordinator.* Introduce yourself to the clinic co-ordinator. Ask permission for your presence and ask if there is anything you need to know. Some clinics require you to sign in, make sure you do this. Do not upset the clinic staff.

➡ *Offer to get coffee.* If you encounter a quiet moment in clinic, offer to get drinks in for the doctors and nurses. It is not a lot of effort and will be well appreciated.

➡ *Ask questions.* Time after time you are advised to ask questions, but there is no better opportunity than in a clinic. Once the patient leaves the room, you are alone with a knowledgeable professional; you can ask questions which may have been inappropriate when the patient was in earshot. You also have time, between patients, to look up answers to questions you asked yourself during the consultation (e.g. in the *Oxford Handbook of Clinical Medicine*).

➡ *Be thorough but concise.* If you are asked to see a patient on your own, do not take the whole clinic doing so. Learn to concisely ask relevant, useful questions.

➡ *Prepare.* Do not go to clinic if you know nothing about the subject the clinic is based upon. Do some prior study otherwise it is a waste of your and the professional's time.

CHAPTER 9

Theatre

What are the different ways you can get involved in an operating theatre? What is expected of you? How do you 'scrub up'? This is an introduction to the etiquette of theatre.

> Arrive at theatres early to leave enough time to find where the scrubs are kept and where to change – staff members are often not happy with you 'popping' in once the surgery has started.
>
> Make sure you know the patient's medical and surgical background – always read the notes and try to see the patient on the ward the evening before they go to theatre.
>
> Know your anatomy – there is nothing worse than being made to feel stupid. (*Kate Fraser, fourth-year medical student, Manchester*)

VITAL STEPS FOR OPERATING THEATRE SUCCESS

These steps must be followed 100% of the time. Before you even step inside an operating theatre you MUST, that is MUST, gain consent from the following people.

➡ *The patient*: ask the patient on the ward, not when they are just about to be put to sleep in the anaesthetic room. Make your function or reason for wanting to attend the operation clear and explain that they can refuse to have you there if they so wish.

➡ *The theatre sister*: the theatre sister rules the operating rooms and will be most dissatisfied if you do not acknowledge this position.

➡ *The consultant*: the patient is under the care of the consultant. Ask his or her permission to be present. If the consultant is not undertaking the operation, also ask for consent to be present from the operating doctor.

➡ *The anaesthetist*: your theatre experience can be greatly enriched by observing and assisting in the anaesthetic procedures and intubation of the patient. If you ask the anaesthetist's consent to be involved before the patient arrives, you may be able to observe and assist in the patient's whole journey from anaesthetic room to recovery.

Take a full history and examine all patients before observing them in theatre. Be familiar with the investigations, especially radiology images (e.g. X-rays, CT scans) as you are likely to be questioned on these in the theatre. Some surgeons will ask medical students to leave if they have not seen the patient or tried to understand the case. You may need to see the patient the evening before their surgery if they have already been admitted as theatre lists tend to start early in the morning.

Try and attend pre-assessment clinics. These are held a few weeks before planned surgery to ensure that patients are fit for surgery and all medical conditions are optimised. Observing explanations of operations for consent purposes will teach you how to phrase information such as medical procedures, risks and benefits. You may be able to practise taking blood and will learn a bit about the patients you will see having surgery in the future.

YOUR FIRST VISIT TO THEATRE

Before you do anything, familiarise yourself with the operating theatre and surrounding areas. Ask one of the nurses or operating theatre assistants to show you around. Specifically, find out:
➡ where to get changed and what to wear
➡ where to stand out of the way but in view of the action
➡ what to do if you do not feel well during the operation
➡ which areas of the operating theatre are sterile.

PREPARATION FOR YOUR THEATRE EXPERIENCE

If you are observing operations from a distance you still need to remove any jewellery and have a good level of personal hygiene. For all trips into the theatre you will be required to wear theatre scrubs (the pyjamas you see surgeons running around in), theatre shoes (clogs) and a hat. Solutions to problems with operating theatre dress, relating to religious practices, can be found in Chapter 13.

You do not usually need your own theatre shoes, spares are often available. Ask which shoes you should use, do not just take any pair.

If you are going to be assisting, or observing the operation close-up, you have to take additional precautions to prevent desterilisation of the operating field. These include the following.
➡ *Wearing a facemask*: doing this is often required even if you are observing from afar; ask theatre staff for instruction.
➡ *Wearing goggles*: usually a case of 'do as they say, not as they do'; you will not always observe goggles or eye protectors being worn; however, in order to

protect you from blood-borne viruses being transmitted by splattered blood wear this equipment.

➡ *Scrubbing up*: a thorough cleaning of the hands, donning a sterile surgical gown and the (near-impossible) task of putting on sterile gloves with (usually still) damp hands; ask for help from experienced theatre nurses. Arrive for the operation in good time so you do not have to rush this step, which can be time-consuming for beginners.

BEHAVIOUR IN AN OPERATING THEATRE

Operating theatre staff and the surgeons work together on a regular basis. When things go wrong, they can go very wrong; this results in a strong bond between the operating theatre staff and surgeons. There may be regular jokes and banter; however, they all know what they are doing and know when this is not appropriate. Do not get carried away with banter or become distracted. If you are asked to assist in theatre give it 100% of your concentration. You will be shown how to hold the instruments in the correct way and you will be told the correct names of the instruments. If you are not paying attention you will irritate the surgeon and may cause a problem.

If you are 'scrubbed up', keep your hands between your navel and your neck and in close proximity to your body until you reach the operating table. You will often see theatre staff and surgeons walking round with their elbows bent and their hands clasped in order to adhere to this requirement. Once you are at the operating table it is often more comfortable to rest your hands on the sterile areas of the table, as directed by the staff.

ACTIVITIES YOU CAN UNDERTAKE IN THEATRE

What you do while you are in theatre will depend on your stage and the surgeon. However, the following activities and clinical skills can be learned and practised in theatre.

➡ *Suturing*: medical graduates are required to be proficient in suturing. The operating theatre is a relatively non-daunting environment as the patient is usually asleep. Real experts, often the theatre nurses, can teach you. The only other clinical environment you can get such good real-life practise of suturing is A&E.

➡ *Examination of patients*: examination of some abnormalities can be easier when the patient's muscles have been relaxed as part of the anaesthetic. However, you MUST gain consent prior to the operation if you plan to examine patients while they are asleep or you could be charged with assault.

➡ *Urinary catheterisation*: patients are commonly catheterised in theatre. You may be less embarrassed to practise while the patient is asleep. However, it must be stated once more that it is ESSENTIAL that you gain prior, explicit consent from the patient for you to carry out this procedure.

WHAT NOT TO DO

➥ Do not act disrespectfully towards the patient. Gain prior consent before laying a hand on the patient while they are asleep. The fact that they do not know what you are doing does not give you the right to do what you like.

➥ Do not get in the way. Operating theatres are generally smaller than those seen on television. It is really easy to get in the way. Be aware of your position and the position of sterile equipment and people at all times. You will become very unpopular if you cause the consultant to have to get changed because you touched them.

➥ Do not undertake any activity that you are not confident to do. Things can go very wrong in surgery. If you are unsure of what is being asked of you or are not confident that you can assist adequately, inform the surgeon immediately. They would rather you asked than made a mistake.

➥ Do not forget about the patient. Visit them after the operation to see how they are getting on. Find out about any problems and look at their notes and drug chart for information on their post-operative care. As a junior doctor it is the post-operative care on the ward that will primarily be left in your hands. Take this opportunity to learn about pain relief and anti-sickness medication. It is also nice for the patient if you show an interest in their recovery.

FURTHER READING

Ng Y. Getting the most out of an operating theatre session. *StudentBMJ*. 2006; **14**: 207.

CHAPTER 10

Community placements

Often sniffed at, community placements can be a rich source of education. So what can be learnt in the community?

Medical students are required to learn about the management of people with recurrent and/or chronic illnesses, mental and physical disabilities and rehabilitation.[1] Community placements provide an excellent opportunity for you to do this. Community placements often, but not exclusively, involve time at a general practice surgery. Therefore, much of the advice given in this chapter relates to general practice placements; although it can be translated or adapted to many other community placement options (e.g. community hospitals).

Community placements may be a solid block of time in the community or one day a week (or month). Experiences will differ depending on the time spent at one placement, but try to integrate into your community teams.

> Community placements offer students an opportunity to see patients' lives in a more complete 'picture'. It can take on many forms, ranging from sitting in a clinic to accompanying the alcohol and drug abuse outreach teams on their visits. There are many opportunities to see how patients adapt to illness in their own homes. You will also get an idea of the role of carers. If you think community placements are boring perhaps you should suggest to your tutor what activities you would like to do to improve them. (*Kate Fraser, fourth-year medical student, Manchester*)

Unfortunately, community placements are often criticised by medical students. Clinical students are familiar with the all too common moans of hospital doctors about general practitioners (GPs). From early on medical students are biased against general practice. However, general practice is a challenging and interesting specialty, and good GPs are worth more than their weight in gold; this is recognised by patients and hospital doctors (if pushed!).

In the early years you will often sit in on consultations with the GPs or the practice nurses. As you progress through your clinical years you are likely to become more independent. However, you will only manage this if you have gained a good insight into the common problems and management of patients in general practice, which are often quite different from those of hospital medicine.

DURING THE CONSULTATION

Presenting complaint – is this the actual problem?

Patients may be embarrassed or worried about the real reason they came to see the GP. Sometimes the presence of a medical student prevents patients from wanting to divulge information about the abnormal growth they have found on their buttock. At other times the patient may be worried their problem is too trivial (or too worrying) to mention alone, so they create a list of problems to bolster up their problem (or delay mention of it). After the patient has left, consider how or if the real problem was mentioned and how different it was from the patient's presenting complaint.

What did the patient want from the consultation?

Patients consult GPs for many reasons; why did each patient come? Diagnosis? An acute problem? Management of a chronic condition? Reassurance? Medication? Sick note? Referral? Company?

How was a management plan reached?

Time constraints may make it tempting for GPs to lead the development of management plans. However, patients are more likely to be satisfied with and follow a management plan developed through a two-way discussion.

Did the patient leave satisfied?

If not why do you think they were not?

Try and think of how you would manage the situation

Were all the important questions asked? If not, why not? Was time a constraint? Thinking of the questions you would ask will prepare you for the GP or nurse turning to you to ask the patient questions. Think of the management options before they are discussed. Was the final plan the same as yours?

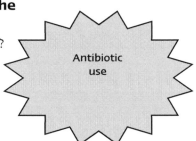

Antibiotic use

AFTER THE PATIENT HAS GONE

Ask questions after the patient has departed if there is anything you are unsure about, or if your question is of a sensitive nature (e.g. you are wondering if the patient has cancer). GPs often know their patients very well and a lot may go unsaid;

without asking questions and resolving unclear information, your experience will be devalued.

Ensure you look up any drugs or diagnoses you are unsure about either between patients, or note them down to look up later on.

WORKING INDEPENDENTLY

Senior medical students can often work independently (space allowing). You may see your own patients and call the GP when you have finished; alternatively, you may be observed conducting consultations. This can be daunting but invaluable. To make the most out of this time try to:

➡ look through the patient's notes prior to them entering the room; you do not have the luxury of knowing the history of many/any of the patients

➡ examine the patients when appropriate

➡ present the patient to your tutor if the consultation has not been observed, include your ideas for further investigation and/or management

➡ try and review patients you see; if you start a patient on a particular medication, ask them to return for review on a day that you will be taking your own surgery again; you will learn how to follow up, manage problems with medication and see the effects of your management plan.

Some of the mundane jobs done by GPs can be useful learning tools. Although not the most interesting exercises, try performing some of the tasks outlined below and you will be surprised how much you can learn from it.

Go through repeat prescription requests. Be thorough. Check requests against all other medication being taken. What are the possible interactions? Are appropriate blood results and monitoring tests up to date? Work out why the medication has been given. Should the patient be on anything else or seen in surgery before the medication is prescribed? Can any of the medications be reduced or stopped?

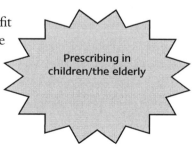

Polypharmacy and associated problems

Go through blood results. Why was the test performed? What action is required?

Take bloods. General practice provides relatively fit patients having routine blood tests. These patients are likely to have good veins and are easy practice for boosting confidence.

Prescribing in children/the elderly

Remember: NEVER change, stop or instigate a patient's treatments. The exercises above are for practice; discuss all cases with the GP.

SKILLS YOU CAN PRACTISE IN THE COMMUNITY

Community placements provide great opportunities to refine your history and examination skills. Time restraints require you to be concise; you only have time to ask about and examine relevant areas. In addition to these general skills, community placements may be the only place you get to witness and perform some procedures and techniques, for example baby checks, smears, dermatology and basic ear, nose and throat (ENT) examinations.

NOT JUST ABOUT GENERAL PRACTICE

The community placement encompasses much more than just general practice, with its GPs and practice nurses. Seek out opportunities to spend time with community midwives, occupational therapists, opticians, pharmacists, social workers, health visitors, chiropodists, specialist nurses and a vast array of other community health professionals. Some GP placements may also offer wider experiences from working in cottage hospitals to general practice clinics in prisons. Even if you do not enjoy the classical GP setting, you are likely to find something that captures your interest and enthusiasm.

FOLLOW UP THE PATIENTS YOU SEE

During your placement(s) in the community you will gain additional benefit from following up some of the patients. Make a list of some of their details (e.g. name, patient number), keep it at the surgery (to protect confidentiality) and look up their details and recent consultations or correspondence when you are next back at the GP surgery. Check any blood test or X-ray results you were involved with ordering and evaluate whether they provided useful information, whether you would do the same again given a similar situation in the future and what more may need to be done. If patients are admitted to your base hospital, try to visit them and follow them up (with their and their consultant's permission, of course).

A FINAL WORD

Like most things in your medical training, the community placements are what you make of them. If you do not make the most of your community time you may get bored, but this is not inevitable. Community medicine is the way forward; procedures and management are increasingly taken out of secondary care and placed into primary care. Without knowledge of the roles, benefits, limitations and problems faced in primary care, you will be ill-equipped to understand and follow the likely future changes in healthcare. In addition, many of you will have a placement during your foundation training in general practice; this will undoubtedly be easier if you have gained a good understanding of community medicine whilst a student. There is much to be learnt, many useful experiences to be had and a real-life view of patients to be gained in the community; undertake your placements with enthusiasm and an open mind and you are likely to learn a lot. Crazy as it sounds, you may even enjoy yourself.

CHAPTER 11

How to get the most from medical school

More than 60 specialties exist in medicine and surgery, each with its own sub-specialties. It is impossible for medical school curricula to incorporate all specialties. Therefore, self-selected components of the course and self-directed extra-curricular activity facilitate further (or new) experience of the specialties that interest you or are an area of personal weakness. So how you do you make your medical training as useful, broad and full of variety as possible?

Optional components of the medical degree may be formally arranged into projects or the elective period (*see* Chapter 12). However, you may wish to undertake additional experience independently. Use your initiative to pursue your interests while you still have the freedom of being a medical student.

SIGN-UPS

'Sign-ups' may be known by different names. Indeed, they may not formally exist. The term 'sign-up' here refers to the process by which you arrange to spend time experiencing a clinical environment or procedure that is different to your official university placement or ward. For example, if your placement is gastrointestinal surgery for a gastrointestinal module, you may wish to complement your learning by watching colonoscopies in the gastroenterology department. You can do this via a 'sign-up'.

To attend a 'sign-up' you must ask permission from your tutor or consultant. You may be presumed to be in bed if you are not on the ward. In addition, it is rude to leave your ward without permission if you are expected to be there.

If there is an official sign-up system in your medical school, use this to book your experience. If there is no official system, telephone or visit the department, introduce yourself and explain what you would like to do. You will often be accommodated, although sometimes patience and flexibility is required.

WORK WITH ALL TYPES OF PROFESSIONALS

Spend time with professionals from each discipline. You can gain invaluable experience from shadowing community or district, primary care and palliative healthcare professionals. You do not need to shadow everyone in every team in which you are placed but do take up relevant and useful opportunities during your clinical years.

Specialist nurses often offer a lot more experience of patient care and their journeys than many other professionals and, as a result, can offer some of the richest educational experiences. Specialist nurses work closely with consultant teams, as well as often visiting patients in the community and running their own clinics or consultations. Specialist nurses often have more time to spend with each patient and this may result in a closer relationship in which patients are more open about their condition and their lives (this also happens because specialist nurses are not doctors!). You will learn about the patient (not just their illness) and how their lives have been affected by their problems. You can still be witness to consultant consultations (for which specialist nurses are often present) and management by other professionals who are involved in the patient's care.

STUDYING ABROAD

The opportunity to study abroad should be open to you; this may occur via your elective (*see* Chapter 12) or you may go abroad to study for a module or a student-selected component (SSC) (*see The Medical Student's Survival Guide 1: the early years*). Your medical school should have a clear policy regarding the availability of the schemes that allow you to do this.[1]

European option

Some medical schools offer a 'European option' for European study. This may require you to already have achieved A-level standard (or equivalent) in a foreign language (usually French, German or Spanish) and/or you may have to attend weekly language classes while at medical school. Depending on your academic record, you may be invited to spend part of the time studying for your course abroad at a European university. Time abroad will usually occur within your clinical years.

Erasmus scheme

'Erasmus' is the 'European Community Action Scheme for the Mobility of University Students' and is the higher education part of 'Socrates', the EU's education programme. Erasmus offers the opportunity, and money, for university students to study for three to twelve months in another country. The Erasmus scheme is open to university students studying any degree for which the Erasmus option is available. To be eligible your university must have been awarded the Erasmus University Charter. Although, for the majority of medical students, the year away in another country may be inappropriate, you may be able to study at an Erasmus university for your elective or SSC and/or as part of the European option that some medical schools offer.

For more information contact your International Relations/European Office about your university's Erasmus links. Try going to the Careerscope website (www.careerscope.info) for information on purchasing *Experience Erasmus – The UK Guide*, which contains information on the degree and diploma courses that can be combined with Erasmus. This guide may also be available at your local school or library. Useful websites include www.erasmus.ac.uk (UK Socrates – Erasmus Council) and www.esn.org (Erasmus Student Network).

EXTERNAL COURSES

External courses are those that have an educational basis but are not part of the medical school curriculum. Many are national and intend to provide you with a deeper understanding and experience of a particular career that you are considering. External courses are often run by the Royal Colleges to promote their own specialties. However, some courses are run by professional organisations and charities. Details of external courses are disseminated by medical schools and journals (e.g. *StudentBMJ*). However, if you have a particular interest, look on the appropriate Royal College and/or organisation websites.

Trauma conference

The trauma conference (www.traumamedicine.org) is a successful external course. Run annually by Bart's and The London Medical School, it is open to medical students nationally. The course occurs in the summer and is aimed at students interested in emergency medicine. General practical skills are demonstrated and taught (e.g. suturing, airway management and spinal immobilisation). More specialised procedures are included as well. In 2006 a trip to a fire station was arranged to teach delegates how to extricate patients from motor vehicles. The three-day lecture and workshop-based conference finishes with a ball, which enables all medical students and course organisers to mingle at a social level. A fee is payable for the course, which is run on a non-profit-making basis. However, past attendees agree it is well worth the money.

FURTHER READING

Killeen T. Travelling man. *StudentBMJ*. 2006; **14**: 154–5. (This article contains useful information for students wanting to study abroad as part of the Erasmus exchange programme.)

CHAPTER 12

Electives

The elective is often the highlight of the medical course for students. How do you arrange it? From where can funding be sought? How can you stay safe? Read on for advice.

Your elective will usually last six to ten weeks and it provides an opportunity to study away from your normal medical school environment. This period is usually incorporated into your penultimate or final year of study. You have total freedom to go wherever and do whatever you want, providing you will be safe and you can illustrate the educational benefit of your choice. Approval from the Dean of your medical school is required before you are allowed to go. Medical student leaders are strong advocates of medical students having the opportunity to study abroad. As a result, travel abroad may occur during your elective, core curriculum study or student-selected components (SSCs; *see The Medical Student's Survival Guide 1: the early years*).[1]

You may dream of what you want to do as soon as you enter medical school. Despite the hours you spend thinking about your options, you may have difficulty deciding what you want to do, where to go or how to organise it. The options open to you for your elective are endless and thus cannot be listed. However, consider the following advice to make planning easier and more trouble-free.

RESOURCES TO HELP YOU PLAN YOUR WHOLE ELECTIVE

Your medical school should give you information on arranging your elective. Records of past students' electives may be held along with information on safety and good travel companies. In addition, you may be able to access health advice if you are going to areas where risks of malaria, HIV/AIDS, or both, are high.

Electives for medical students

The British Medical Association (BMA) Medical Students Committee has published guidance, *Electives for Medical Students*, to assist you in planning your elective. The guidance is available to members free of charge from askBMA (0870 606 0828). Further information can be found on the BMA website (www.bma.org.uk).

Medics Travel

Medics Travel (www.medicstravel.co.uk) is designed for doctors, nurses and healthcare students who want to plan work or electives with overseas hospitals, non-governmental organisations and charities. Medics Travel contains updates for the book, *The Medic's Guide to Work and Electives around the World*.[2] You are invited to submit information on your own elective when you return, with the chance of payment if it is published.

Medical Defence Union

The Medical Defence Union (MDU) (www.the-mdu.com/ten) offers its members 'The Electives Network' (TEN). TEN is designed to make elective planning easier by providing information on medical schools and hospitals across the world. It contains a funding database and has links to flights and an accommodation provider. A free guide to planning your elective, the *MDU Guide to Electives*, is available to members via the website. The MDU website contains articles that cover important topics such as research and planning, where to go and what to do as well as travel information.

Medical and Dental Defence Union of Scotland

The Medical and Dental Defence Union of Scotland (MDDUS) (www.mddus.com) has produced an elective booklet that contains guidance and hints for planning your elective. It is relevant whether you are planning your elective in the UK or abroad. There is also some information on sources of funding. The booklet is free to MDDUS student members and can be obtained via the website.

HOW TO CHOOSE WHAT TO DO

Make a careful, considered decision about your elective. It must:
➡ benefit you educationally
➡ provide you with the experiences you desire
➡ enable you to have fun and be safe.

Start planning early on. It takes a long time to decide on what you want to do, plan it, book it (including the accompanying insurance, accommodation, etc.) and undergo any vaccinations you may require.

What are you interested in?

Is there a specialty you are interested in undertaking as your future career, but you have not yet had enough experience to commit yourself? Do you want to see how the developing world manages with even less money than the National Health Service? Maybe you are interested in non-mainstream branches of medicine (e.g. prison medicine)? If any of these apply to you, use your answers as a basis upon which to start looking for an elective.

Destination

Any elective experience is highly personal. Some students see it as the last opportunity they have to travel for a significant number of years. Other students have no interest in 'widening' their medical education by getting gastroenteritis. There is an unspoken competition among medical students to go to the most far-flung places. Do exactly what you want to do with this time. Do not feel ashamed if you are not travelling thousands of miles.

> I had a fantastic time on my elective in Dublin. I experienced the relatively unknown world of forensic psychiatry. I was worried before I went that I was only going to Ireland, but I was getting married four weeks after I returned so I did not want to be far from home in case of problems (and I did not want to be away from my fiancé for the whole eight weeks). I had never been introduced to forensic psychiatry before I went, and it was so vastly different from anything I had ever done before that I could have been on the other side of the world. Being near to home also meant that my fiancé could come to visit for the weekend every two weeks and I had no problems with language. *(Lizzie Cottrell, fifth-year medical student, Manchester)*

You may not mind what you do providing you can go to a specific destination. If this is the case, *The Medic's Guide to Work and Electives around the World*[2] is an invaluable resource. Each chapter is dedicated to a different country and/or city. It provides details of hospitals, clinics and local information. The beginning of the book also contains useful general advice on planning an elective.

If you do not know what you want to do or where to do it, consider the following questions and see if they direct you to a country, or at least a continent!

- Do you want to stay in your home country or go abroad?
- Do you have financial responsibilities that you do not want to compromise?
- Do you have children or dependants that you want to be near?
- Is it likely you will need to come back and re-sit an exam?
- Are you an international student?
- Have you considered returning to your native country to reduce expenses?
- Do you want to experience a different culture? Different cultures exist even within one country. However, huge differences in culture exist all over the world. Have a think about the type of culture you want to experience; start by choosing between developing and developed countries.
- Can you speak foreign languages? It is bad enough being in foreign country when you are on holiday if you are not fluent in the local language. Things get a whole lot worse when you add medicine into the equation.
- Do you want to be linked to a medical school? The benefits of being linked to a medical school in your destination are that you may receive teaching and

be able to organise accommodation. However, the downside is that it restricts potential destinations. Even if a medical school exists, it may not be interested in forging links with you. See the details on the Institute for International Medical Education (IIME) website (www.iime.org) for details of how to contact medical schools around the world.

Think of a few destination options in case your first choice does not work out; it may be too popular, too expensive or too dangerous. You may only be allowed to travel to one destination unless a proven additional educational benefit is gained by multiple stops. Do not set your heart on 'travelling around Africa' until you have checked with your medical school whether this is allowed.

Websites that may help you decide where to go

The BMA website for medical student electives (www.bma.org.uk/ap.nsf/Content/electiveguide) contains information provided by past students. A printable document, the *Elective Guide*, is also available at the website. Both the website and the document provide information that includes details and advice on how to get to a number of countries, accommodation and past experiences.

The *StudentBMJ* website (www.studentbmj.com/international/international.php) provides reports from previous students' electives. The information is divided into continent and country groups allowing easy access. Visit this for more information to help you decide where to go.

The Institute for International Medical Education (IIME) is responsible for the development of 'global minimum essential (core) requirements' required of doctors throughout the world. IIME also collates global information on different aspects of education in the medical profession. The IIME website (www.iime.org) contains a database of medical schools across the world, which contains addresses and websites, searchable by content and country. There are also links to popular medical journals and organisations from around the world.

Work the World (www.worktheworld.co.uk) is a website that provides healthcare students with high-quality, supported overseas placements. *Work the World* also arranges group projects to enable students to tackle globally important issues (e.g. HIV/AIDS, malaria). You will have to pay for a placement; however, you get a lot of experience and support for your money.

FINANCES

Finances may be a major restriction. Electives can be expensive. Once you have decided what you want to do for your elective, investigate the cost of the following.

➡ *Travel to your destination*: if you are likely to want to return home, multiply this appropriately.
➡ *Accommodation*.

➧ *Food*: if your destination is remote and does not produce much of its food and drink, costs will be increased for shipping.
➧ *Health*: do you require vaccinations or anti-malarial prophylaxis? Do you have to pay for any of this? Post-exposure prophylaxis kits can be invaluable in HIV-prevalent areas but are expensive.
➧ *Travel insurance*: do not skip this to cut costs.
➧ *Transport*: is your accommodation near to where you will be working? How are you going to commute? How much will this cost?

Once you have worked out the likely cost of your elective, work out if the funds you have are enough. If not, read on, other sources of financial help may be available.

Sources of help

You may be able to obtain financial support from a number of sources:
➧ loan: you may be of the mindset that your elective is a one-off opportunity and you do not mind how much it costs; after all, you will be earning within the next year; if this is the case then taking out a loan may be an option for you
➧ scholarship
➧ bursary
➧ sponsorship
➧ competition prizes
➧ parents or family.

Some sources of funding are only provided for electives undertaken in certain specialties. Others require you to undertake specific research projects during your elective. Competitions are usually essay-based on a subject relating to the specialty to which the providers of the prize are related.

Websites to assist with finding funding for your elective

The BMA medical student web page (www.bma.org.uk/ap.nsf/Content/Medical electivescontactinfo) provides a directory of sources for funding an elective. The directory provides details of the type of funding, quantity, application requirements and contact details.

The MDU runs a competition for its members to win a substantial sum of money towards an elective. You have to answer a few, simple questions before the annual deadline. It is well worth visiting the website (www.the-mdu.com/ten) for more information; you never know, you might just get lucky.

The MDDUS administers the charitable organisation, the British Medical and Dental Students Trust (BMDST). The BMDST offers scholarships to medical (and dental) students who are taking their electives abroad. Up to £600 is awarded. For further information on application information and deadlines visit the website (www.mddus.com).

ARRANGING YOUR ELECTIVE

> There are amazing things to do if you get in there early enough flying doctors in Tanzania and the Australian Outback are not impossible placements to get if you apply a couple of years in advance. *(Kate Fraser, fourth-year medical student, Manchester)*

Make provisional enquires and applications at least one to two years before you are due to go. Unfortunately it is not always possible to find out from your medical school when you will be going on your elective this far in advance. However, you can make provisional enquires whilst pushing your medical school to tell you when your elective will take place as early as possible.

Book your transport in advance. This is often the most expensive part of your elective. First try a student travel centre (e.g. STA travel; www.statravel.co.uk) to see what deals are available. Alternatively, price comparison (e.g. www.cheapflights.co.uk) or the Association of British Travel Agents (www.abta.co.uk) websites may be useful. Be aware that some budget airline companies have very low luggage limits. If your luggage is over the weight restriction, the excess must either be removed or paid for by the kilogram; this can soon add up.

Booking accommodation in advance can be difficult. This is anxiety-provoking as your elective draws nearer and you still have nowhere to stay. Try local university accommodation, ask your contacts at your elective destination (e.g. hospital accommodation, friends with spare rooms, etc.) and try websites which advertise rented properties. Private rented accommodation may only be advertised a month in advance if this is the notice the current tenants are required to give before they leave.

ENSURING IT ALL GOES WELL

Travel insurance

Travel insurance for your elective is essential. Do not neglect it or you may regret it. Some general holiday travel insurance companies will not provide the cover you require on your elective. Thankfully, medical student elective tailored insurance can be obtained.

Whatever policy you take out, check that it is valid for your entire trip and that it covers all the people who are travelling. Be clear about what is covered in terms of activities and luggage. Check exemptions carefully and make sure you have told the insurance company about any pre-existing medical conditions that you have. Do not forget to take with you the policy number and emergency telephone number and leave a copy at home.[3]

British Medical Association Services

British Medical Association (BMA) Services (www.bmas.co.uk) offers travel insurance designed to meet the needs of medical students going on their electives. The insurance covers needlestick injuries, emergency medical expenses, personal belongings and liability, repatriation expenses if you need to return home for medical treatment and cover for portable medical equipment. An important consideration for some is that it covers cancellation in the event of exam re-sits.

Wesleyan Medical Sickness

Wesleyan Medical Sickness (www.wesleyan.co.uk/doctors/medicalstudent/travelinsurance_3091.html) offers medical student elective travel insurance. It covers cancellations for exam re-sits and adventurous activities and portable medical equipment. In addition, Wesleyan Medical Sickness offers inclusive personal accident cover in the event of an HIV needlestick injury. Further details on this cover can be found on the website.

Medical indemnity

Make sure that you have medical defence cover. Placements will often require evidence of your indemnity cover and some countries or areas may prevent you from obtaining full indemnity (e.g. Australia); clarify these points early in your elective planning process. If you have indemnity with a UK company, you may be able to avoid paying for indemnity cover at your host institution.

In general, your indemnity cover may only be provided if your elective has been authorised by the Dean of your university, is properly supervised by a qualified healthcare professional and does not exceed your qualifications.

Medical Defence Union

The Medical Defence Union (MDU) (www.the-mdu.com) offers free indemnity cover for your elective. In addition to this, members have access to a 24-hour advice line for medico-legal issues. Discretionary assistance is available for claims arising from Good Samaritan acts performed anywhere in the world. Just tell the MDU your destination and, in return, they will send you written confirmation of your indemnity cover. If you are undertaking your elective in Australia, the MDU will not provide indemnity for you; however, the helpline and cover for Good Samaritan acts is still available.

Medical Protection Society

The Medical Protection Society (MPS) (www.medicalprotection.org/medical/United_Kingdom/) provides indemnity and advice for its student members on elective (in most cases). A 24-hour emergency telephone advice line provides support and advice through (actual or potential) ethical or legal dilemmas. The cover also provides assistance with claims arising from Good Samaritan acts occurring anywhere in the world. If you are planning to travel to Australia send an e-mail to elective@mps.org.uk to ensure you are properly protected.

Medical and Dental Defence Union of Scotland

The Medical and Dental Defence Union of Scotland (MDDUS) (www.mddus.com) will provide free indemnity to its student members for their electives. If you are a student member of the MDDUS you should contact the Membership Services Department and let them know where and when you will be doing your elective.

Visas and passports

Make sure you apply for a full 10-year passport and/or visa in plenty of time when needed (see the website www.passport.gov.uk). Such documents take some time to be processed. If you already hold a passport, check that you have more than six months left before its expiry date (many countries insist on this). Find out if you need a visa to stay and/or work during your elective from a travel agent or from the Consulate or Embassy in the UK of the country you are going to travel to.

Make sure you have written the details of your next of kin in the designated space at the back of your passport.

Ethics

Electives in developing countries often appeal to students wanting to do more than they can do in their own country. However, even if it is offered, do no more than you are allowed to do at home (e.g. prescriptions).[4] The patients you are looking after are not guinea-pigs. It is unethical to view such people as subjects on which you can practise skills you are unqualified to do at home. Concentrate on the other benefits of an elective in a developing country. There is an increased need for accurate clinical judgement as a result of reduced availability of tests and investigations, and conditions often present in later, more advanced stages as patients do not have the resources or education to seek help earlier.[5]

Safety

Although you can use your elective to gain experiences of cultures and environments that are totally different to what you are used to, do not jeopardise your life or safety (see the Suzy Lamplugh website for more advice; www.suzylamplugh.org). Some areas of the world are volatile. Undertake risk assessments with your medical school prior to your elective; assess violence, political instability and likelihood of natural disasters.[4] To gain current, updated advice and information on the area of the world you would like to travel to, visit the Foreign and Commonwealth office website (www.fco.gov.uk/travel).

Do not take anything valuable with you unless it is absolutely necessary. Traveller's cheques can reduce the amount of cash you carry; just make sure you write down all the numbers and put them in a separate place while you are away, and leave a copy at home. Do not carry large amounts of cash; only take out what you need for the day. Leave extra cash or traveller's cheques in a safe, if available. If you are taking debit and/or credit cards (check they will not expire while you are away), make sure you also leave one in the safe. Make a note of your card details and contact numbers and keep these details separate from the cards (and leave a copy at home) just in case they are lost or stolen. Invest in a money belt for secure and secret possession of money. Take copies of your passport, insurance details and travel documents, and keep these separate from the originals.

Certain areas of medicine can be more dangerous as a result of blood-borne diseases. Therefore, carefully consider the risks of undertaking obstetrics, accident and emergency or trauma work in an area with a high prevalence of blood-borne diseases.[6]

HEALTH

The Department of Health website (www.dh.gov.uk/PolicyAndGuidance/Health AdviceForTravellers/fs/en) offers advice for travellers.

Common things are common

Eating freshly prepared, hot food in areas of poor sanitation can prevent diarrhoea and vomiting. Avoid uncooked vegetables. Fruit can be eaten, providing it can be peeled. Only drink bottled water or tap water that has either been boiled or sterilised. Avoid ice in drinks if you do not know the source of water that has made it.

Coughs, colds and flu can occur at any time so they may occur while you are away. It is difficult being ill while you are away, but treat yourself in just the same way as you would at home. Stay at home if you are too ill to attend your placement. Drink plenty of fluids and rest. If your symptoms are severe, or unlike any other previous cold/flu you have had in the past, seek medical attention, especially if you are in a tropical climate.

Heat stroke and sunburn are real risks when working in a hot climate. You will not be accustomed to the intense heat that occurs in some favourite elective destinations. Protect yourself against dehydration by drinking large quantities of clean water, use a high factor sunscreen if you working outdoors and stay out of the sun when it is at its strongest.

The fact that you are travelling does not make you immune from accidents. In addition to cuts and scrapes, traffic accidents are very common among travellers. Be careful when out and about in foreign countries.

If you have a pre-existing medical condition, make sure you have adequate medication to last for the duration of your trip. Pack the medication in its original packaging along with prescription documentation. Some medications may be illegal in other countries. If you are taking medications with you, check with the Embassy of your destination that they are acceptable and/or whether you also require a doctor's letter.

Communicable diseases

Sexual health may be an important consideration for some. Whether you are male or female, take condoms with you. If sexual relationships are a possibility, carry condoms with you at all times. Do not rely on unknown foreign brands. Be careful, you are vulnerable, especially if travelling alone. If you go back to a new acquaintance's house, your sexual and physical safety is at risk.

Take care in clinical environments at all times. Regardless of the sophistication of the healthcare system you should do this anyway. However, some areas of the world have a high prevalence of HIV; needlestick injuries in these places are far more likely to result in serious problems. Before you go, assess the risk that communicable diseases pose in your proposed destination.[4] Weigh up if you think this risk is acceptable against the benefits of carrying out your elective in this environment. (See this website www.doh.gov.uk/traveladvice.)

Post-exposure prophylaxis

If you are travelling to an area with a high incidence of HIV, prepare yourself for the unfortunate event of a needlestick injury (*see* Chapter 13; *see also* the website http://hivinsite.ucsf.edu/international/) from an HIV-infected patient. Take with you post-exposure prophylaxis (PEP) drugs to provide you with the best chance possible of preventing the disease occurring. The best results from post-exposure prophylaxis occur if the drugs (anti-retroviral therapy; ART) are given within hours of exposure to HIV.

You may be travelling to a remote or poorly funded area for your elective; do not rely on being able to obtain effective medication soon enough after your exposure. Before you travel, ask your university or local communicable disease consultant for information on the most appropriate ART treatment to take with you. Obtain clear instructions as to when you are required to take PEP.

PEP is taken for four weeks after the exposure to HIV. However, the drugs have significant side effects; these can be so severe that they may prevent you from continuing to work while you are taking them.[7]

Malaria

Malaria is treatable and preventable but potentially fatal. Find out if your elective destination requires you to take anti-malarial medication. If prophylactic medication is required, take ALL of it. The prophylactic drug you require depends upon the risk your destination carries, the extent of drug resistance, side effects and any other health conditions you have.[6] Consult your GP for the most appropriate anti-malarial medication for your circumstances.

In addition to anti-malarial medication, additional precautions will reduce the risk of malaria. Invest in a good mosquito net; nets that are impregnated with permethrin are best. Make sure this totally covers your bed area at night with no gaps. Other useful protective methods include coils or vaporised insecticides, roll on/spray/lotion insect repellent and long-sleeved/legged clothes to wear after dusk.

Vaccinations

The need for vaccinations before you embark on your elective depends upon where you go. If you are travelling to Australia, Europe, New Zealand or the USA you will not require any special immunisations. However, make sure that your childhood immunisations were completed and you have been immunised against tetanus and poliomyelitis.[6] If you are travelling to Africa, the Middle East, Asia, South America and some areas of the Mediterranean,[6] visit your GP at least six weeks before your departure to book and obtain the vaccinations you need. Some vaccinations carry a fee; budget for this when planning your elective. (See these two websites: www. thehtd.org and www.fitfortravel.scot.nhs.uk.)

Local problems

Wherever you plan to go, find out local information. What is the prevalence of HIV/AIDS? Are there poisonous animals, fish and plants? Is it a malaria risk zone? Is the tap water safe? If not, where can you obtain bottled water? If you believe you are going to an area in which the water is not drinkable, make sure you take some sterilising tablets. Plan on preventing local health problems from developing, rather than on having to deal with them.

Medical equipment

Medical equipment may be required should you become ill while you are away. If you take your own, you can be assured of the hygiene and quality standards you are used to in the UK. It is recommended that you take the following equipment:[8]
➡ injection or venepuncture equipment: syringes, needles, intravenous cannula
➡ suturing equipment: needle and silk, skin closing strips
➡ dressings
➡ alcohol swabs
➡ disposable gloves
➡ medications: do not take anything that is illegal at your destination; however, in addition to taking your regular medications, take some basic medications such as paracetamol and ibuprofen in case you get a minor ailment.

European health insurance card

The European health insurance card (EHIC) has taken over from the old E111, as a means of getting free or reduced cost emergency care if you are travelling within the European Economic Area or Switzerland (See the websites www.ehic.org.uk and www.dh.gov.uk/travellers.) The EHIC is issued free of charge. You will still require travel insurance to cover things that the EHIC does not (e.g. repatriation to the UK), and some travel insurance policies may not be valid without the EHIC.

Take a copy of your EHIC with you and leave one at home in case the original gets lost while you are away.

WHAT TO DO WHEN YOU GET THERE

Do not forget that you will not be spending 100% of your time at your placement. You are going to have free time. Get your hands on guidebooks, brochures and website information to find out how to make the most of being a tourist.

Local customs

Make sure you are aware of local laws and customs. In particular, find out about appropriate dress, alcohol laws and use of cameras or binoculars around military sites or airports. You will be working with the 'locals' and you may offend them by not complying with local customs (e.g. greetings). The following websites offer guidance: www.brookes.ac.uk/worldwide; www.lonelyplanet.com; www.tripadvisor.com.

FURTHER READING

Department of Health. *HIV Post-exposure Prophylaxis: guidance from the UK Chief Medical Officers' Expert Advisory Group on AIDS*. London: Department of Health; 2004.

USEFUL WEBSITES

www.bba.org.uk (Contains information on using your credit cards abroad.)
www.oanda.com (Contains cheat sheets for foreign currency exchange values.)

CHAPTER 13

When things go wrong

Go ahead and take risks. Just be sure that everything will turn out OK.[1]

It is perhaps a surprise that this chapter is not entitled 'If things go wrong', but this would be a falsely optimistic title. Medical school is tough and there will be times, for everyone, when things go wrong. Read on for advice on some of the more common problems that you may face while at medical school.

WHAT TO DO IF YOU HAVE A PROBLEM WITH YOUR MEDICAL TEAM

Throughout your time as a medical student you will encounter many healthcare professionals and, inevitably, this will present a problem at some stage. Indeed, healthcare staff members encounter many medical students and may have had problems in the past, thus they may be weary of you. Be aware of the problems that may occur through working in a medical team and learn how to deal with them.

Personality clash

You will never get on with every member of every team. If you appear to be having a 'personality clash' with another team member, first make sure you are not:
➡ being bullied or harassed
➡ bullying or harassing your team members
➡ being oversensitive.

If the above are not applicable, find ways of completing your placement successfully. If your issues are with another medical student, can you separate and work in different areas? Could one of you go to clinic while the other is on the ward (swapping intermittently)? If you have a problem with a doctor or nurse, can you work with another? Have other people had the same problem? What did they do?

Sometimes compromise and reluctant acceptance is required to avoid jeopardising your learning. This can be stressful so make sure you can let off steam in a safe, professional and constructive manner.

> Harassment is unwanted conduct that violates a person's dignity or creates an intimidating, hostile, degrading, humiliating or offensive environment having regard to all the circumstances and the perception of the victim.[2]

Bullying and harassment

Bullying and harassment are serious issues. They can make your immediate life a misery, increase your risk of alcohol misuse and depression,[3] and affect you in the long term by reducing your confidence and enthusiasm for training. Thankfully, many medical students report that they have never been a victim of bullying and harassment. However, 20% have experienced bullying and harassment infrequently and 2% experience these unacceptable behaviours at least monthly. The most common forms of bullying and harassment towards medical students are verbal abuse and exclusion, most commonly by doctors and nurses.[4]

Although it found bullying and harassment to be relatively uncommon, nearly half the cases of bullying or harassment that occur are not resolved. In the majority of cases in which resolution occurred, it resulted from the actions of medical students themselves.[4] If you are being bullied know your rights and act in accordance with them.

Who is bullying you?

Doctors are the main perpetrators of bullying towards junior doctors in training, with nurses and midwives also being a significant source of negative behaviour.[5] Nobody has the right to act negatively towards you. If you are being bullied it is wrong. Act immediately to stop the perpetrator and to protect your self-esteem. Seek advice from university or hospital staff, friends and family.

> . . . [clinical] experience without training increases confidence not competence.[6]

Inadequate educational input

Doctors are busy with clinical responsibilities and a life away from medicine. You are not the number one person in their lives and their input into your education may not be recognised. However, they should be willing to undertake teaching.[7] Therefore you should expect teaching on your clinical placements. If you are consistently failing to receive teaching, think of reasons that may explain this and devise possible solutions.

Are too many medical students present on the placement? Organise your time-tables together so you split up to ensure only one or two students attend each place at any one time. Do not split up for teaching sessions (unless they are practical ones) so the doctors only need to cover each topic once and can thus cover more topics.

Are you expecting too much? Is your tutor actually meeting the requirements but not going any further? If so, you may not be getting as good teaching as your peers, but if your tutor is not fulfilling expectations then you have to seek help, education and experience from another source. If your tutor does not fulfil their role, inform your medical school.

Who is responsible for your teaching? Find out who is the named person responsible for your teaching and speak to them. They may have delegated the job to another individual who is shirking their responsibilities.

Is your placement busy? Formal teaching will suffer in busy environments. Patient care comes first. Immerse yourself in ward life and get as much 'on the job' teaching as you can. Ask questions when appropriate and you will learn huge amounts.

RESTRICTION OF RELIGIOUS PRACTICES

> From 2 December 2003, when the employment equality (religion or belief) regulations came into force, it became unlawful to discriminate against workers because of religion or similar belief.[2]

> The GMC has not published any guidance which specifically addresses the issue of medical students or doctors wearing face veils. We do have a policy to promote equality and value diversity. We do not set out guidelines about the dress that medical students should or should not wear . . . graduates can obtain registration . . . providing that they can meet the outcomes set out in *Tomorrow's Doctors* and are fit to practise to the standards set out in *Good Medical Practice*. We do not consider that wearing a face veil, in and of itself, necessarily has any effect on a doctor's ability to practise medicine. However, good communication between patients and doctors is essential to effective care and relationships of trust, and patients may find that a face veil presents an obstacle to effective communication.[8]

Medical students come from many religious backgrounds. This diversity contributes to a rich education surrounding multi-faith societies. However, it can lead to specific problems. You must make sure you are not unfairly discriminated against. Many of the barriers to your religious practices that medical school may hold can be overcome and should not prevent you from getting an adequate education or experience.

Many medical students have not been discriminated against because of their culture, and the majority do not think religious beliefs disadvantage students.[4]

Medical schools are also supportive of students who need reasonable time out of education for religious occasions. However, for a minority, problems do occur. Some basic examples of religious-based problems, specifically relating to being a medical student, are outlined, but general specific advice cannot be given here as acceptable solutions vary from university to university and hospital trust to trust.

Depending on your religion and/or religious practices, restrictions or problems encountered at medical school may include accommodation of specific dietary requirements, easy access to places of worship and disagreement surrounding suitable attire or medical practices in clinical areas and/or theatre.

Increasingly, medical students are assisted to practise their religion appropriately and fully without having to miss out or avoid educational experiences. Universities have chaplaincies that offer support, places of worship and information on the world's major religions, and many hospitals provide a number of places of worship for the main religions. Medical degree courses have incorporated cultural diversity into the curriculum to improve acceptance and understanding among the student population, this benefits students and patients.[9]

Some hospitals provide sterile over garments to be worn in theatre over a *hijab*; others allow students to take in clean headscarves or to have specific theatre headscarves; check with theatre staff at your hospital(s). Large surgical hats or orthopaedic surgical caps (helmet-like opaque caps) often cover headwear (e.g. turbans, *hijab*, *kippah*) and may be an easy and acceptable solution for some. Similarly, theatre scrubs that are felt to be too revealing can be worn with a theatre gown over the top to provide a high front and long sleeves. Some hospitals have theatre scrubs in the shape of a dress; these can be worn over trousers.

Canteens are recognising the need for choice and, depending on demand, the need for certain preparatory practices. Groups and societies have formed within universities to gather together all followers of the same religion. These act as social support and sources of information and solutions.

Unfortunately, some medical students have come across fundamental problems relating to their religious practices which have not been overcome satisfactorily. Adequate policies are not in place and/or standardised across the country for every issue that arises; solutions found in one hospital may be totally unacceptable, inappropriate and/or impossible to implement in another. Even within hospitals, accepted practices may not always be agreed to by each member of staff, thus creating interpersonal conflict in the clinical environment. Structural and procedural problems can create restrictions of religious practices within the hospital; for example, 'scrubbing up' (thoroughly washing hands and arms) before theatre involves exposure of the arms in communal areas. Some Muslims would find male and female scrubbing areas a more acceptable solution, but this is likely to be impossible unless it is considered during the construction phase of new facilities. One solution to this problem is to wait until everyone else has scrubbed up before you do the same, thus giving you private space.

The concept and practice of abortion is emotive within religious and non-religious groups. If you do not agree with abortion (or contraception) you are within your rights to not be involved in the procedure; some doctors will not refer for or perform abortions for religious reasons. Explain to your tutors that you do not feel you can be witness to the procedure and they should understand this.

Decide by yourself, or with the help of family members or religious instructors, what is and is not appropriate within your religious practices. Be clear on what you can and cannot do, then be open with your university. If you need to take time away for religious festivals or occasions, give plenty of notice and either make up the time or obtain the missed work, as appropriate. Similarly, expect your university to be open regarding policies (e.g. dress codes) and helpful in providing possible solutions. If examinations fall on a festival or religious observance day, you may be able to sit the exam at an earlier time than the rest of your peers. Ask your university if teaching sessions can be changed if they regularly conflict with prayer times. Contact your university's international office or your medical school tutors if you encounter seemingly insoluble problems or restrictions that relate to your religious practices.

Guidance and information relating to religious practices and the workplace can be found on the Advisory, Conciliation and Arbitration service (ACAS) website (www.acas.org.uk). Lastly, if you have been subject to non-medical school-related racism- or religion-based threats or crime, inform your university's welfare officer and/or the police as appropriate.

> When the student qualifies it will almost inevitably be necessary to put patient care before religious observance on occasion. At some point, therefore, the aspiring doctor has to choose to put their patients before their religious observance. Ultimately, patient care must come first, and with this in mind, we need to try and strike a delicate balance.[8]

ASSESSING AND MANAGING DETERIORATING PATIENTS AND EMERGENCIES

Identifying, assessing and managing deteriorating patients and emergencies are not your responsibility as a medical student, but they will be as soon as you qualify. Deficiencies in the initial assessment and treatment of acutely ill patients on wards by junior doctors lead to unnecessary death.[10] Get as much experience as possible in these skills, and make sure they are second nature by the time you qualify. Although this section introduces emergency assessment, you must get

Pulse oximetry

official training and practise before you qualify. This is literally a life-or-death subject that must not be taken lightly.

The Resuscitation Council has introduced the idea of the 'chain of survival' (Figure 13.1).[11] Each link of the chain is equally important and essential in the successful care of a severely ill patient. Learn how to identify, assess and manage patients at each link of the chain before you qualify.

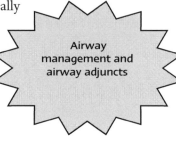

Airway management and airway adjuncts

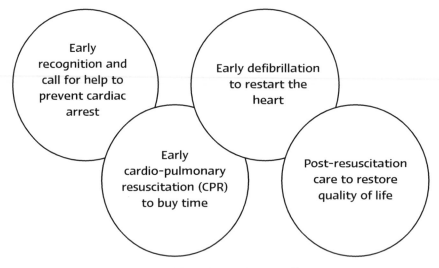

Early recognition and call for help to prevent cardiac arrest

Early defibrillation to restart the heart

Early cardio-pulmonary resuscitation (CPR) to buy time

Post-resuscitation care to restore quality of life

Figure 13.1 Resuscitation Council (UK) chain of survival.[11]

Outcome following cardiac arrest is unfavourable for most patients. Pre-arrest care is thus becoming the main focus of advanced life support (ALS) and should be high on your learning agenda to increase patients' survival and quality of life. The widely used 'ABCDE' (airway, breathing, circulation, disability and exposure) approach to emergency assessment is used repeatedly throughout the pre-, peri- and post-arrest situations. This is the most appropriate order in which you should approach the assessment of an acutely ill patient. Find out what assessments, normal values and actions are taken at each step of the ABCDE approach.

While you are at medical school, try and observe as many cardiac arrests as you can. Help by inserting cannulae and taking arterial blood gases. If you are trained, you may be able to ventilate the patient and perform cardiac compressions. DO NOT get in the way at an arrest. Every second counts. The experience you gain as a student in an arrest situation is invaluable; the environment is like no other.

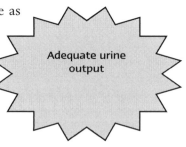

Adequate urine output

Even if your patient is resuscitated successfully, the healthcare team cannot relax. The hard work is only about to start for the patient, who is critically ill and at risk of arresting again. Post-resuscitation care is crucial to recovery and discharge. It starts when spontaneous circulation is restored within the patient; the patient may still not be breathing independently. Learn about post-resuscitation care, including methods of oxygenation, post-arrest investigations, optimising organ function and the management of post-resuscitation complications.

You will receive training directly through your medical school for basic and advanced life support. Courses, aside from the medical school curriculum, include the Advanced Life Support (ALS) course and the Acute Life-threatening Events Recognition and Treatment (ALERT) course. Attend these courses if you get the chance. Run by experts, they are very informative. You will get lots of practise and alleviate some uncertainties. Learn about the ethical issues surrounding resuscitation, which can be a minefield and an area of conflict once you start work.

COPING WITH PATIENTS DYING

Unfortunately, patients die – even after faultless care. This is a harsh reality of life. You need to accept and cope with this. As a junior doctor you will be expected to verify and certify patients as dead.

Exposure to death is variable throughout medical school. If your course includes dissection, you will be introduced to a room full of dead bodies very early on. When entering clinical placements exposure to death can occur anywhere: in the GP's surgery; on the ward; in an operating theatre; and in non-university-based situations, such as in a shop or the death of a friend or family member. Exposure to death can both desensitise and heighten your emotions surrounding death and dying. You become aware of the unfairness, sadness and relatively short nature of human life. Monitor your responses towards death and dying, and speak to friends, family or tutors if you are struggling to manage your emotions.

Emotions, reactions and attitudes to death

Normal emotions, reactions and attitudes to death vary between people or from situation to situation.

➡ *Grief and sadness*: especially if you knew the patient or they were a friend or family member. Sadness ensues to some degree in most deaths; you feel sad for the family, that the patient did not have a family and just because a person has died. It is OK to demonstrate sadness to friends and the relatives of the deceased (they may even find reassurance in this), but do not get into a situation in which they have to comfort you.
➡ *Relief*: occurs as a result of a cessation of the suffering you have seen the person go through before their death. Try and focus on this positive outcome if you are upset.

➥ *Anxiety*: especially during your first exposure – you may be unsure what a dead person looks like. This is often overcome quickly on the first exposure when you realise there is nothing to worry about.

➥ *Lack of breathing*: strange as it sounds, there is often an overwhelming awareness that the person is not breathing.

➥ *Calm*: can ensue, especially after deaths that have been the result of a failed resuscitation attempt or an unpleasant terminal event (e.g. massive haemorrhage).

➥ *Disappointment or frustration*: may be felt if you have been involved in the care or resuscitation of the deceased.

➥ *Questioning of own religious beliefs*: regular exposure to death makes life seem vulnerable and short. It seems unfair that nice and/or young people die. Seek support and advice from your usual faith leaders. Try to understand why a death has happened or find peace in yourself about the death. Such support may also be found from your university or hospital chaplaincy.

➥ *Rumination*: some deaths are forgotten by home time, others play on your mind and a week later you realise you have gone over it repeatedly in your head. Take time to think about why you keep pondering the death. Are you upset? Are there uncomfortable issues surrounding the death? Speak to someone you trust. If you are upset about specific issues regarding the patient, speak to an involved staff member in an attempt to resolve your feelings and accept the death.

'Do not resuscitate' orders

Death does not only occur because the medical team has not done enough. Failures in healthcare do exist; however, often death occurs because nothing more can be done. It can be cruel to fight this natural process. If intervention is likely to be futile, and (importantly) the patient agrees, your goal should be to maintain comfort and dignity. In these circumstances 'Do not resuscitate' (DNR), 'Do not attempt resuscitation' (DNAR) or 'Not for resuscitation' (NFR) orders are placed in the patient's notes (the terminology is interchangeable). DNR orders may be implemented if the patient expresses their informed wish not to be resuscitated if they undergo cardiac arrest even if you believe it not to be futile.

DNR is not synonymous with no further treatment. In many cases you should continue to do all you can to treat the patient with a view to cure unless instructed otherwise by the patient. Palliative care is the main exception, as the focus is on symptom relief rather than cure.

MISTAKES

You are only human, thus mistakes are inevitable. Just do your utmost to be safe and thoughtful. Be accountable for all of your actions, including making mistakes. There is a line between mistakes and negligence; be sure you do not cross this.

Avoiding mistakes

Although you will make mistakes, you can reduce the number by following a few simple steps.

➥ *Do not work beyond your means.* Your medical school should provide guidance on what you are and are not allowed to do as a medical student. In addition, you know what you can do and what you cannot; thus judge if you are capable of doing what has been asked of you. If you are in any doubt or feel unsure do not continue.

➥ *Ask if you need help.* Nobody minds you asking (unless you have asked the same question hundreds of times previously), especially when the alternative is that you do something wrong. Just make sure you are asking questions at an appropriate time and do not continue with your intended activity until it is totally clear in your mind what you are doing and why.

➥ *Get supervision.* If you have not carried out a procedure before (or are still not confident), ask for supervision. Your tutors may have to pick up the pieces if you do something wrong, they would much prefer to supervise you than undo the mess you have made.

➥ *Ask for fully informed consent from the patient before performing procedures.* Ensure you ask the patient's permission once you have explained what you are going to do. The act of explaining the procedure to the patient will confirm that you know what you are doing, how you are going to do it and why you are doing it.

➥ *Document what you have done.* The documentation process should be thorough. Take time to think about the details of what you have just done or are about to do. This can help to order your thoughts and may trigger you to realise you were about to miss/have missed something and prevent a mistake from happening.

Medical students and mistakes

The mistakes of medical students should not be serious as you cannot undertake dangerous procedures or decision-making without supervision. You are usually accountable to your tutor (e.g. consultant, GP) and/or medical school. However, you still must behave professionally and within your limitations.

When you become a doctor you will be required to follow the guidance '*Being Open*' (available from the National Patient Safety Agency). This document instructs healthcare professionals to tell patients why, what and how a mistake was made, and to express sympathy and regret (but not admit liability). Remember these points when patients are talking to you. Medical students are often a sounding board for patients who are dissatisfied with a service or individual and who are victims of mistakes. Use these experiences to learn how to manage negativity without getting individuals into trouble or fobbing the patient off.

If you have made a mistake, admit to it promptly. Tell a healthcare professional, your tutor or your medical school as soon as you can. Mistakes should be identified and investigated for teaching or learning purposes (not just for discipline). Many people may learn from your mistake; without you making others aware the same mistake may be repeated. Honesty and bravery in owning up to a mistake should be commended. Learn to face up to your actions before you become a doctor.

NEEDLESTICK INJURY

'Needlestick' injuries refer to injuries arising from needles or other sharps, such as surgical instruments, bone fragments and glass vials. The problem with such injuries in the healthcare setting is that they carry a risk of transmission of blood-borne viruses.

The risk of transmission of blood-borne viruses depends upon the nature of the exposure (e.g. puncture of the skin), the body fluids involved (e.g. blood, amniotic fluid, semen), the infectivity of the patient and the nature of the injury (e.g. deep injury from a hollow needle carrying blood).[12]

How to avoid getting a needlestick injury

Follow protocols, involving sharp disposal and use of sharps, in order to prevent needlestick injuries when performing procedures. Dispose of sharps immediately as you finish with them at the point at which you used them (i.e. take a sharps bin to the bedside). Do not ask others to clear up for you; they may forget and it puts them at unnecessary risk. Conversely, medical students are not there to clear up other people's sharps when you are observing them. Being unsure of how many sharps have been used results in the risk of an incomplete collection; thus causing a future risk of a needlestick injury. If you see a sharp that is unprotected in a clinical area, do your best to dispose of it safely; ask if you are unsure how to do this.

Avoid re-capping a needle. If you absolutely have to replace the cap use a one-handed technique. Lay the cap down on a flat surface and let go; then introduce the needle into it.

Sharp instruments, needles and equipment must not be disposed of in a plastic bag, but in a hard plastic container. You will find these clearly labelled around all clinical areas of hospitals, clinics and GP surgeries. If you are unsure how to dispose of an object correctly ask a trained member of staff. You may not only be putting yourself at danger, but also others, including porters, nurses and the general public, if you throw things away in the wrong place.

What to do if you get a needlestick injury

Make sure you know the recommendations for dealing with a needlestick injury in your hospital. You may be advised to squeeze the area to encourage bleeding and wash the wound with soap. Report the injury immediately to a senior doctor or nurse and occupational health.

Local pain and infection following a needlestick injury are a concern. However, the main concern is whether you have contracted a serious communicable disease from the sharp that has entered your skin. Such diseases mainly include HIV, hepatitis B and hepatitis C. The risk of getting HIV infection from a needlestick injury is <1%.[13] The risk of transmission of hepatitis B ranges from 6% to 40% depending on the infectivity of the patient, determined by markers in their blood.[14] The risk of transmission of hepatitis C after needlestick injury from a patient with hepatitis C infection is between 0% and 7%.[15]

A blood sample from the patient involved in the use of the sharp may be required to determine whether they carry a serious communicable disease. For this you *MUST* gain informed consent. If the patient is unconscious their blood cannot be tested until they have regained consciousness and given their consent. If consent is not given, or is unlikely to be available in the next 48 hours, you and your occupational health advisor should calculate your risk of infection. You may be required to take medication 'just in case'.[16]

If you have an unconscious patient's blood for a diagnostic test do *NOT* use it to test for a serious communicable disease unless you have sought advice from a medical defence organisation as you may be liable for prosecution. If you go ahead and use this blood to test for a serious communicable disease, inform the patient at the first opportunity. Results of the test must not be entered into the patient's medical notes without consent following testing that occurs in this manner.

FURTHER SCENARIOS

You will find advice on the following situations in *The Medical Student's Survival Guide 1: the early years*:

➡ bad days
➡ failing exams
➡ dropping out of medical school
➡ support for medical students
➡ fitness to practise.

FURTHER READING

Department of Health. *HIV Infected Health Care Workers: a consultation paper on management and patient notification*. London: Department of Health; 2002.

Grant P. Dealing with dying. *StudentBMJ*. 2003; **11**: 260. (A really thoughtful insight into the reality of death to medical students and junior doctors.)

Liverpool care pathway: information on care of the dying. (Available from: www. lcp-mariecurie.org.uk)

Palliative care resources (Available from: http://book.pallcare.info; http://palliative

drugs.com; www.ncpc.org.uk; www.palliative-medicine.org; www.palliative carescotland.org.uk)

Tagal J. Don't talk about death: we're medical students. *StudentBMJ*. 2006; **14**: 78–9.

CHAPTER 14

Difficult individuals

One doctor's list of difficult patients is not the same as another's.[1]

Doctors usually work closely with the public. Inevitably you will be in contact with 'difficult' individuals. Why are people 'difficult'? How do you best manage 'difficult' individuals? Finding an answer to these questions as a medical student will reduce the chances of your working life becoming a miserable battleground.

WHY ARE INDIVIDUALS 'DIFFICULT'?

Dealing with 'difficult' patients, friends and relatives (individuals) is unpleasant. It is estimated that such patients comprise 15% of the clinical practice of doctors.[2] So what causes individuals to be labelled as 'difficult'? Some seem not to want to help themselves, some want to help too much. Their priorities may differ from your own. Rudeness or aggression can occur with or without unreasonableness. Many factors act upon patients, their friends and their relatives during illness. Only by recognising these may you appreciate that 'difficult' behaviour may be an understandable response (Figure 14.1).

To cope with 'difficult' individuals try to understand their situation. Run through the items in Figure 14.1. Can the individual's behaviour be explained by any of these? Do not forget, patients are often told bad news in an unfamiliar environment; this may have greater psychological and emotional effects than you may appreciate. Many patients have underlying social problems and these, rather than medical problems, may cause the most difficulty.

The media is often guilty of 'doctor-bashing'. Doctors are often made out to be incompetent, uncaring and more interested in going home on time than patient care. As a result, the general public's attitude is increasingly negative towards doctors, hospitals, nurses, medical students and other healthcare professionals. Negative attitudes can manifest during admissions and consultations. Healthcare professionals thus need to put greater effort into gaining the respect and trust of patients. Some patients may never trust you, so convinced by media 'evidence' they interpret any explanations to the contrary of their beliefs as a fob-off or a cover-

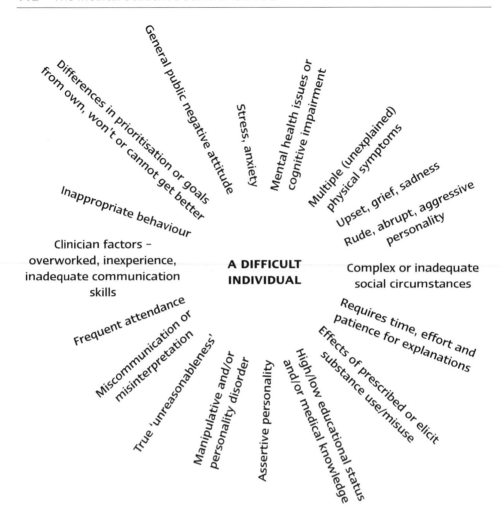

Figure 14.1 Possible factors leading to an individual appearing 'difficult'.[2]

up. Trust is so important in doctor–patient communication that a patient with a negative attitude is truly 'difficult'.

Stress, anxiety, upset and grief can manifest in various ways; for example, anger, irritation, impatience, denial, seclusion and irrationality. Individuals sometimes react in a 'difficult' way when told bad news or when coping mechanisms fail. Rather than being labelled as 'difficult', such people require extra time, understanding and support.

Individuals under the effects of prescribed, legal or illicit substances can become irrational or disinhibited. Similarly, some mental health problems or cognitive impairment may result in an absence of abstract thought processes or an inability to problem-solve. This can make communication, diagnosis and management difficult. Often, third parties are involved with such patients (e.g. friends, relatives, carers, social support services). The 'difficulty' arises because management is not straightforward. Usually the most 'difficult' components of management are access to adequate funding and willing professional input. However, with the right people good management will happen.

Some individuals are 'difficult' (or frustrating) because they do not seem to look after themselves. Patients may smoke, drink or eat to excess; they may do no more exercise than going to the toilet or ignore all prescribed medications. However, as healthcare professionals your function is to *advise* and *educate* – not to dictate the way people should live their lives. Every individual you meet has different priorities to you. Provided that they are armed with and understand all the facts, learn to respect their choices.

You may find yourself labelling individuals as 'difficult' when they are too pro-active with their health. Often holding high educational status, such individuals spend a lot of time researching their ailments on the internet, take numerous self-prescribed complementary remedies, or both. Complementary therapy does have uses and can be beneficial; however, it presents 'difficulties' when patients do not know what they are taking. Some complementary substances interfere with 'traditional' medical treatment and may be toxic. Autonomy boosts self-esteem and increased feelings of control over health and well-being. However, the danger with self-diagnosing, self-medicating individuals is that they convince themselves of their diagnosis and then only present the relevant symptoms to you. This can bias the consultation and potentially mask other (more accurate) diagnoses.

'Difficult' patients may only be so to you as a result of a personality clash. Some people may be inherently rude, abrupt, aggressive, assertive or 'unreasonable'. Only experience and professionalism will help you to handle such patients.

Some patients may be judged as being 'difficult' because they present 'a challenge'. Real, insoluble problems that cannot be managed any better are out there. You have to learn to accept that some patients will have a poor quality of life and are in a difficult situation. Do not neglect such patients: maximise their care and provide them with support; do not allow your frustrations to be reflected onto them.

COMPLICATIONS OF THE LABEL 'DIFFICULT'

The label 'difficult' can stir up negative feelings within you. These can include anger, anxiety, frustration and defeat.[2] This may result in avoidance behaviour: you and other healthcare professionals may avoid any unnecessary contact with that individual. This is damaging to the patient's care and may even worsen the situation.

Some 'difficult' individuals pose a real danger to health professionals. Individuals who are prone to violence, verbal abuse or unfounded complaints can damage the body, mind and reputation of all the professionals involved in their care.[2] If you have internally labelled a patient as 'difficult', assess any risks they present. If you believe the patient poses a risk, seek help from your seniors on how to handle the individual.

A vast amount of time is spent working with 'difficult' patients. Complaints may be numerous, and each one requires investigation. Placating individuals when they are highly stressed can take time, and you will spend a lot of personal time reflecting on the uncomfortable situations that accompany difficult individuals.

HOW TO MANAGE 'DIFFICULT' INDIVIDUALS

As with any healthcare professional, medical students should not tolerate abuse or violence. If you are exposed to threats or any uncomfortable situation (e.g. raised voices) leave calmly and inform another healthcare professional.

No responsibility for care or management falls on a medical student's shoulders. Therefore, if you find patients or their relatives 'difficult' you can choose to avoid contact. However, unless there is a risk of a complaint, avoidance is not helpful in the long term. Learn how to manage such situations to prepare you for when you qualify. Observe how existing doctors deal with difficult individuals. However, some situations may be unsuitable for you to witness; respect this, your patient's care is the priority.

Be alert to internally labelling individuals as 'difficult'. Your attitude towards such patients must remain professional and normal. Exercise extreme patience, even if you have to vent your spleen to the healthcare staff involved afterwards. If an individual is acting unreasonably (but does not appear to pose a risk to you) deal with them in a firm, caring and non-confrontational way. Outline the limits and expectations of reasonable behaviour.[2]

The label of 'difficult' often stems from problems with communication and misinterpretation of information. Be proficient in effective communication and discuss management plans clearly. Try to talk to as many patients as possible. Some patients are more willing than others to converse with you in wards or clinics; however, make the effort with them all. This will build your confidence, provide you with techniques in gaining rapport and teach you how to change your communication approach to suit the patient.

Ask your medical school to incorporate 'dealing with difficult individuals' into your communication skills sessions.

Constructive discussion with peers and colleagues, without breaking confidentiality, will help you to reflect on your experiences and gain advice for future management. Expert psychiatric opinions can be of use in those 'difficult' individuals you believe to have mental health problems.[2]

If you are really struggling with 'difficult' individuals, look to your own attitude and behaviour. Could you be perceived as a 'difficult' individual? Excessive arrogance and poor communication skills can really damage potential relationships and rapport with patients. Individuals may act in a 'difficult' way because they cannot relate to you.[2] If you are not coping with the workload or work environment your communication skills and attitude may suffer. Look after yourself and seek help and support if you start to feel things getting on top of you.

CHAPTER 15

Life after medical school

> At times, the thought of your own career in medicine can be analogous to the contemplation of outer space . . . too immense to comprehend.

CAREER PLANNING AND ADVICE

Career advice and counselling is a major part of the 'Modernising Medical Careers' (MMC) initiative. You require structured career support as you are expected to make important decisions about your future career in your second postgraduate year.

Good and appropriate career advice should be available throughout your training and career. Medical schools should incorporate preparations for job applications (e.g. CV design and interview skills) as part of the curriculum.

The assessments that occur throughout medical school will help you with career decisions. They will highlight your strengths and weaknesses, likes and dislikes, and areas requiring further development. The more seriously you take these assessments, the easier career decisions will be to make.

You are responsible for your own career development and pathway. If there is something you feel the medical school should provide, request it. Such resources may include career fairs, workshops on interview skills or development of career forums.

POSTGRADUATE TRAINING

Postgraduate medical training has become more streamlined and standardised since the MMC initiative. However, important career decisions have to be made earlier than in previous postgraduate training schemes. Figure 15.1 illustrates the MMC career framework, from medical school through postgraduate training to a specialist or general practice career. Further information on postgraduate training, careers and the MMC initiative may be found on the MMC website (www.mmc. nhs.uk). An interactive version of the career framework diagram may be found at www.mmc.nhs.uk/pages/interactive-diagram.

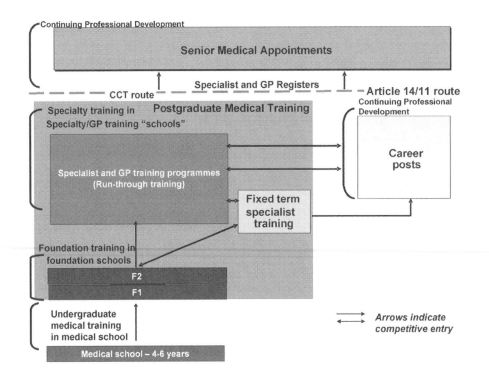

Figure 15.1 UK Modernising Medical Careers (MMC) career framework, 2006.

Foundation programme

The Foundation programme comprises the first two years after graduation from medical school. These years are called Foundation Year 1 (FY1) and Foundation Year 2 (FY2) and have replaced the House Officer (HO) and Senior House Officer (SHO) posts, respectively. Unlike the previous system, if you successfully complete the FY1 year you are guaranteed an FY2 post in the same area.

The Foundation programme was designed as part of the MMC initiative to ensure quality and safety in doctors. It is a structured and assessed programme that all medical school graduates must enter and complete successfully before embarking on general practice or specialist training. Unlike the old scheme for junior doctors, Foundation doctors have regular workplace-based assessments of clinical and non-clinical competences which are based on explicit criteria laid out in the Foundation curriculum.[1] The General Medical Council (GMC) and the Postgraduate Medical Education and Training Board (PMETB) have agreed the curriculum. From 2007, the GMC will only award full registration if all outcomes required from the Foundation curriculum are achieved.[2]

In order to progress through the Foundation programme and into GP or specialist training, you will need to maintain a national learning portfolio.[3]

The Foundation programme posts have been designed to encourage medical school graduates to experience a wide range of specialties. Not only does this include more obscure careers but less popular ones ('shortage specialties'), such as academic, teaching and research careers. Increased experience is achieved by rotations involving three posts per year (rather than the old system which included two) and taster opportunities (up to a week out of study leave in FY2 year to spend time in a specialty of interest).

Run-through specialist or general practice training

Before the MMC initiative, you had to pass the relevant Royal College membership exams to qualify for specialist or general practice training schemes. Revision for these exams cut into your junior doctor training. Since the MMC initiative, the Royal College exams are no longer entry criteria for further training, nor are research degrees (unless you want to go into academic medicine). This allows you to concentrate on meeting the requirements of the Foundation curriculum.

Applications to run-through specialist or general practice training schemes occur during Foundation training and are extremely competitive. Specialty or general practice training programmes start immediately after successful completion of the Foundation programme. If you are working in a career post, fixed-term specialist training post or other run-through specialist or general practice training programme, you, too, can compete for the run-through specialist or general practice training schemes.

The length of the specialist training after the Foundation programme is usually between five and seven years. General practice training usually lasts for three years. The run-through specialist or general practice training programmes are based on, and assessed in accordance with, a curriculum agreed by the PMETB. The run-through specialist training programmes start by being broad-based, for example core medicine or surgery. As you progress through the specialist training you narrow your field to your desired specialty. Make a decision about your career to enable you to direct your training appropriately.

If you complete a run-through specialist or general practice training programme successfully you will be awarded a Certificate of Completion of Training (CCT). With a CCT under your belt you are eligible to apply for senior medical appointments such as consultant or general practice principal posts.

Fixed-term specialist training posts

Fixed-term specialist training posts are open to doctors who have successfully completed their Foundation programme, but who do not have run-through specialist or general practice training posts. These are hospital-only posts, and contracts are for a maximum of two years. Re-application must occur annually, either for run-through training or for another fixed-term specialist training post.

Fixed-term specialist training programmes reflect the first two years of a run-through specialist training curriculum. However, further training is unavailable in a fixed-term specialist training programme. If you take up a fixed-term specialist training post owing to an unsuccessful application to a run-through specialist or general practice training programme, work hard to improve your application. Re-apply to a run-through specialist or general practice training programme as soon as possible.

If you are not interested in the specialist or general practice training programme, or have repeated unsuccessful applications, you may apply for a career post. These are service-delivery posts, that is, your job is to provide care to patients not to further your training towards being a consultant. In order to become a consultant or general practitioner (GP) from a career post, you would generally be required to apply and successfully complete the run-through specialist or general practice training programme (even if you have spent years in fixed-term specialist training posts or career posts).

PREPARATION FOR JOB APPLICATIONS: YOUR CAREER COUNTDOWN

> Always remember you are unique, just like everyone else.

Career countdown

Early preparation is the key to a successful career. Tough competition lies ahead. You must make yourself stand out from everyone else (who are all trying to doing the same). Preparation for your future career should start as soon as you enter medical school; details for this early stage can be found in *The Medical Student's Survival Guide 1: the early years*. This section details the actions you can take to prepare for your applications to your first job.

Early clinical year(s)

Your early clinical year(s) should be relatively stress-free. If you have limited experience of a clinical environment and communicating with patients it can be daunting, but little is expected of you except that you remain professional. Use this time to master patient communication and basic clinical skills in different settings.

If you are offered clinical Student Selected Components (SSCs; *see The Medical Student's Survival Guide 1: the early years*) use them to experience and develop skills in different environments. SSCs may assist you to refute, introduce or confirm a particular area of medicine as your potential future career.

Plan your elective (*see* Chapter 12) as early as possible; ideally one to two years before you go. Consider options that involve experiences, skills and environments that are different to those you have in your normal clinical placements. What really interests you? You will not get many similar opportunities with such freedom again.

Start thinking ahead to your postgraduate, Foundation programme rotations. Which geographical area will you want to undertake this training in? What working environment do you enjoy? Which particular area best caters for the career you want to pursue? Most students are influenced by the location of their medical school and family when deciding where they are going to apply for postgraduate jobs.[5]

Remember that job applications open early in your final year at medical school (usually around October), so start collating evidence that supports the fact that you will be a good doctor. Did you create a Record of Professional Development (ROPD) in your early years at medical school? Has it been updated with skills, achievements, personal qualities and aspirations? Following the recent changes applicants often feel that the Foundation Year application forms do not provide enough space to fully represent themselves.[5] Although application procedures may change further over forthcoming years, try to get one step ahead by planning what evidence you will provide. Note down your major achievements and qualities, and alongside these explain how each will assist you in your future career. Start this early and you will have plenty of time to ponder on good ways of presenting the information about yourself in a clear and concise way.

Refine your earlier career plans, taking into account your increased experience. Do you still want to follow the same career? If you want to be a surgeon, what sort of surgery do you enjoy? Have you realised that working with patients is not for you and laboratory work would be better? Do you want to combine research or academia with another specialty?

Final clinical year

Use your final clinical year to practise being a doctor. You are safe in the knowledge that you have not got many responsibilities . . . YET. Shadow the junior doctors more than the consultants. Learn what their duties are and how to overcome common problems and difficulties. Every time the doctors do something, ask yourself 'Could I do that?' If the answer is no, rectify this.

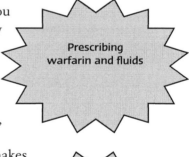

Prescribing warfarin and fluids

Knowing exactly what being a doctor involves makes job applications easier. You will know which skills you require so will make the links between your interests and your future job more obvious.

Put all the skills you have learnt over the past few years to good use. In order to make the most of your final year, be prepared to put in the hours. Do not run yourself into the ground, especially if your final

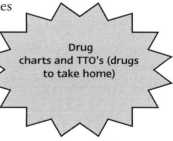

Drug charts and TTO's (drugs to take home)

examinations are looming, but do not expect everything to happen between the hours of 9 am and 5 pm.

Keep your eyes and ears open for career fairs and attend them when possible. National (e.g. BMJ careers fair, National Medical Careers Show) and local (medical school or postgraduate deanery based) career fairs exist for your benefit. Try and attend at least one career fair during your final year to ensure you are equipped with the information you need to follow your intended career path or to assist you if you are undecided on your future. (See these websites for more information: www.medicalcareersshow.com; www.bmjcareersfair.com.)

It is crucial that you continue activities away from medicine. Ensure you have an effective way to relax and distract yourself from work, especially during exam time. Relaxation skills are essential when you embark on your new career; stressful times as a doctor are not far away. Non-academic interests are also a strong feature of the application forms for Foundation training.

Discharge documents

Phone and bleep systems

Completing a certificate for registration of death and when to refer deaths to the coroner

Applying to the Foundation programme

Postgraduate job application procedures are highly controversial. For example, the press coverage surrounding the Foundation application procedure in August 2006 harshly criticised the process when 10% of students were not allocated places on the first round. You have to remember there is no perfect job application process. To be fair, it must be as transparent as possible, that is, it must be clear how a decision to employ or not to employ was reached. Despite the complaints, the job application procedures in 2005 to 2007 were more transparent than the old, interview-based system.[6] Take national media coverage with a pinch of salt, such stories are often fuelled by emotion and contain only limited truth. Keep updated with the real facts and information by visiting the British Medical Association (www.bma.org.uk), Conference of Postgraduate Medical Deans (www.copmed.org.uk) and Postgraduate Medical Education and Training Board (www.pmetb.org.uk) websites. What follows is a general overview and advice about Foundation job applications. Current details must be sought at the time you apply as changes are going to continue until relative satisfaction ensues.

The process in brief

The system used for applications

A centralised Foundation programme application system was introduced for the August 2007 posts. This most recent application system was web-based and UK-wide (see the websites: www.bma.org.uk; www.copmed.org.uk; www.pmetb.org.uk; www.mmc.nhs.uk (includes links to the useful leaflet, *How to Apply Online*); www.nes.scot.nhs.uk/sfas/). Centralised application systems have the advantages that there is less effort involved for students, less time out of studies for interviews, it is fairer and meets equal opportunity legislation, more applicants will be allocated jobs first time round and it is efficient.[7]

Regular changes to the application process make it difficult to offer specific, long-standing advice; however, the information given below is likely to be of use no matter what changes occur in the future. Make sure you read all available information and use the 'help' functions of the online application system to ensure all the information you submit is appropriate and accurate.

What are you applying for?

Those applying for August 2007 posts, will be initially applying to the Foundation schools; each school consisting of a number of institutions (acute and mental health trusts, general practices, universities and so on), grouped together to provide complete and wide education and training. For 2007, students have to rank all 27 UK Foundation schools in order of preference. This system vastly reduces the chances of you not being allocated a job but results in the possibility that you may be placed in an area miles away from where you would ideally like to be.

Think about the following: 'Where is my first-choice area to work?' Think about distance from friends, family, partners and dependants. Are you hoping to buy a house? What is the local area and property market like? How big is each deanery, thus how far may you have to travel within each? Which places lend themselves to your hobbies?

Details of the Foundation schools and details, and estimated numbers of posts or programmes and local students, were available for the first time for the 2007 intake during these initial stages of the application to inform these choices. You will also be able to look at the rotations each Foundation school offers. This stage of the application process usually occurs between October and December, the year before you are due to start.

Once you have received confirmation that you have been accepted into a Foundation school and have received information on that Foundation school (via e-mail in February) you will also be provided with your application score. Now you have to apply for particular posts within your Foundation school. Use your score, as well as your interests, to inform decisions when applying to individual posts (i.e. do not apply to competitive posts if you have a low score). The result of this application process will be available in the March of the year you will start.

Academic ranking

Your medical school will provide Foundation schools with information on your academic performance and any areas of concern, 'ranking' you based upon academic achievement. In addition, it will confirm your eligibility to apply. If you have 'special circumstances' that result in you needing to stay in the area, your medical school will submit this information at the same time.

Outside interests

Information on your interests away from medicine will be requested in every job application you make in the future. Medical students (and doctors) do not have a lot of spare time after they have completed a full schedule in university (or work) and study (continuing medical education) in the evenings and weekends. In addition, financial pressures may result in some medical students using time out of university to work to earn some money.

Do not neglect your university work for time on the football pitch. However, you should master the art of juggling extra-curricular activities with your studies in order to present yourself as a well-rounded individual on job applications. If you have not yet reached your final year at medical school and do not have any real outside interests, try and find something fast. When learning something new, or undertaking a new activity, think about the skills it provides that will assist you in your future career.

Selling yourself appropriately

It is not good enough to write how good you are and all the fantastic things you have achieved if you do not link this information to your future career. Link every piece of evidence you give to how this will make you into a good doctor. Do not assume that the link is so obvious that you do not need to state it explicitly. It is not a matter of what your interests or achievements are, but how you relate them to your future career.

Never lie on any job application. If you think laterally and deeply enough you will be able to think of qualities, achievements and experience you have that you can link to your future jobs. Ten per cent of Foundation programme applications are randomly selected for audit. If you lie or plagiarise on your application form you could be prevented from ever starting your career.

Be clear and concise. The number of words allowed for each statement is limited and important information can be diluted in waffle.

Achievements

A misconception among medical students is that the word 'achievement' is synonymous with 'award'. This is not the case. If you are asked to state your achievements, do not just think about prizes or awards but also about personal achievements; things you are proud about or factors that make you stand out from the crowd. You may have climbed Mount Everest; this, by anyone's standards is a huge achievement, but you may not have received a medal for doing so. Obviously this is an extreme example: a more realistic achievement may be that you have completed medical school and brought up two children. Doing this demonstrates fantastic organisational ability, an essential quality of a junior doctor.

Interviews

The selection process in the years preceding and including 2007 had evolved to exclude interviews. This causes great controversy because applicants:
- may not speak English and will be employed
- feel unable to express themselves adequately or convey essential information
- enter their new jobs 'blind' as they have not had any opportunity to ask questions or meet future colleagues[8]
- may find sources of 'good application answers' thus undermining the whole scheme.

The controversy surrounding the lack of interviews may result in the interviewing process coming back into favour in the future. However, the arguments against an interview in the application process include:
- some evidence suggests that interviews encourage 'like-by-like' selection[9]
- interviews fail to filter out those who are not fit for the purpose[9]
- communication and language skills of potential doctors can be tested by the trust in an informal way.

There is no perfect selection process – what ever method is used or is not used will be criticised by some. You will have to investigate at the time of your application whether interviews are a likely option. If so, make sure you prepare thoroughly for the process. Preparation should include the following.
- Investigate the hospital / deanery / Foundation school to which you have applied. Be able to justify the reasons why you are applying to that institution. Talk to current FY1s to gain an understanding of their roles, responsibilities and working conditions.
- Know your application form inside out. You may be asked to expand on any point you made in your application to date.
- Keep up to date with basic ethical issues and the GMC guidelines, *Good Medical Practice*.[10] You may be asked to demonstrate that you hold the qualities required of doctors that are set out in this publication.

GRADUATION

Graduation with your medical degree represents the confirmation that you are fit to practise to the standards set out by the GMC in *Good Medical Practice*.[10,11] In order to change your name from Miss / Mrs / Mr to Dr on your bank and / or driving licence details, you may require a validated copy of your graduation certificate so keep it safe (this is the only evidence of your qualification). After your graduation you will be provisionally registered with the GMC. You have to pay a fee for provisional registration (£100 in 2006). In order to fully register with the GMC you must successfully complete the Foundation Year 1 post.

Alumni associations

As graduates, you and your peers become alumni to your old university. As an alumnus you are entitled to join the appropriate alumni association; membership is usually free and life-long. As a result you will be provided with means to keep in touch with other alumni, receive invitations to reunions and have access to some university facilities. Other benefits are on offer, and these vary with each institution. To find out more, visit the alumni page of the relevant university's website.

SURVIVING LIFE AS A JUNIOR DOCTOR

> Often the doctor will be the 'new' member of the team left to struggle with the complexities of working with 'a more junior' team member who has better knowledge of the team goals than themselves. Rapid changeover of doctors leaves little time for relationship-building among team members.[12]

After five years' dreaming about this day you wake at 4 am, early in August, with a cold sweat. Overnight you have made the transition from 'ex-medical student on holiday' to 'doctor', on the front line of the fight against death and disease. Worry not; there are plenty of things you can do to make the move as smooth as possible.

Get to know your terrain: shadowing

Near the end of medical school you undergo a period of 'shadowing', or consolidation. This usually lasts from one to four weeks, during which time you 'shadow' the HO/FY1 you are taking over from in your first job. During this period of time, pick your predecessor's brains and do as much as you can to achieve the following objectives of the period.

➡ Find out who is on your team and what the weekly activities of the firm are (e.g. theatre lists, clinics).

➡ Discover your consultant's likes or dislikes. Best to find out now if he insists on daily stool volumes!

➡ Get to know the staff on the ward, not just the doctors.

➡ Find out the ward layout and security codes.

➡ Familiarise yourself with request forms for investigations, know where they are kept, what information is required and who you have to give the completed request to.

➡ Find out and practise the daily activities of your predecessor. For example, filling out drug charts and prescribing warfarin may throw up questions if you have not done it properly before. Discover you are not confident now, rather than when you are alone on the ward.

➡ If the previous HO/FY1 has left you a handover sheet with a list of all the patients, try and get hold of it the day before you start.

Keep track of your patients

At all times, know the names and locations of the patients under your care. This is especially vital if your firm has patients on many different wards. It is embarrassing (and frustrating) when you miss patients out on the ward round and get bleeped at a quarter to five to come and review them. Unless you have a photographic memory, you will need to keep some sort of list. Ways of doing this include the following.

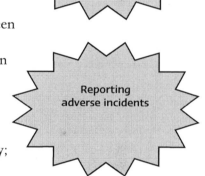

➡ *Computerised printouts*: most hospitals have a facility for printing out lists of the patients under each consultant or ward. Print a new list every morning. Beware: lists are not always completely up to date and may not include all new admissions or patients who have recently been transferred to your care.

Prescribing controlled drugs

➡ *Word-processed list*: keep a crib sheet of patients on a computer and update the list daily with new admissions and jobs to do. A popular method but sometimes time-consuming.

Reporting adverse incidents

➡ *Hand-written list*: may be updated during the day as new patients appear but can quickly get untidy; which results in jobs being missed.

Any list that you use should contain the patient's name, ward, hospital number, date of birth, diagnosis and any jobs relating to that patient which need to be done. Be REALLY careful with any list such as this that you are carrying around. DO NOT lose it; it contains confidential information that can be harmful, embarrassing and unethical if it lands in the wrong hands. When you have finished with the list make sure you shred it or dispose of it in 'confidential waste'.

Carry supplies

Carrying around your own supplies of assorted forms and request cards saves a lot of time and also means that you can fill out the forms on the ward round as an investigation is requested. You may also have nowhere very accessible or secure to store your personal items, such as money, credit cards and keys; think about where you can put these when deciding what to use to carry around supplies.

Common methods for carrying around supplies include using the following.

➡ *Folders*: these have the advantage of providing a surface you can lean on when you write and you can put dividers inside for the different forms. Annoyingly, they take away a spare hand.

➥ *Bags*: these free up your hands and can contain reference books, purse, car keys and snacks; however, you may find carrying around a bag cumbersome.

A typical day in the life of a house officer/FY1
Ward rounds

Most days start with a ward round. Be punctual. If your ward round starts at 9 am be there early to make sure all the required information is available and in the correct place. You will be expected to lead the doctors to the correct patients and update the team with the patients' conditions. Your senior colleagues will instruct you as to what management is required. Write a record of these requests in the patient's medical notes (*see* 'Note-keeping' below) and carry out the plans as appropriate.

Local industrial-related diseases

Doing your own ward round

If a consultant or registrar ward round is not occurring, you will be expected to do the ward round by yourself. Don't worry, you will not be expected to make major management decisions. The aim of these junior doctor ward rounds is to identify any new problems and patients whose condition is worsening or becoming unstable.

One way of organising your thoughts and questions during a self-led ward round is the 'SOAP' method.

➥ *S – Subjective*: How does the patient feel today? Example note entry: 'feels well, ate all three meals yesterday'.

➥ *O – Objective*: Check the observation chart and the urine output. Examine symptomatic patients for any new signs. Example note entry: 'Appears well hydrated, blood pressure 120/80 mmHg, pulse 80 beats per minute, urine output 2000 mL over past 24 hours, fluid input 2500 mL over past 24 hours'.

➥ *A – Assessment*: Write down your overall assessment of the patient's condition today. Example note entry: 'Progressing well post-operatively, wound non-inflamed'.

➥ *P – Plan*: Your plan for the rest of the day. Address old issues that have not been resolved, signs of deterioration and new problems. Example note entry: 'Monitor fluid balance, if vomits again prescribe anti-emetic (anti-sickness drug)'.

Jobs

During the ward round you will develop a list of jobs that must be done to manage the patients. It is tempting to disappear to the doctors' mess for a cuppa but first get the urgent jobs out of the way; you never know what may arise next.

Ordering investigations

Try to fill in the investigation requests during the ward round and then take them to the appropriate place straight after the ward round. Try to get your requests in before some of the other firms. If your team requests an urgent investigation, find out when they want it. Can it be left a few days or must it be done today? Find out the reasons why it is urgent, how will it change the management of the patient? Armed with all this information, go to the appropriate department and speak face-to-face with the appropriate person. You may have to fight your patient's corner and bargain with the department to get the required investigation done in the timescale that you need it.

If you have ordered an investigation, it is your responsibility to obtain the results. Note down pending investigations on your job sheet and only cross them out once the results are written in the medical notes. The best time to set aside for collecting investigation results is last thing in the afternoon and/or when you are doing your own ward round. The latter approach takes longer but allows you to review the patients with the most recent investigation results in mind. If you are waiting for radiology or pathology reports, which can take a while to come through, note down your efforts at chasing the results to ensure it is clear that they have not been forgotten.

If you are working on a Friday, make sure that requests for weekend blood tests are written. There is usually a designated place to leave pre-dated blood forms to ensure the tests are performed on the correct day. Ask the nursing staff about this when you start.

Organise blood results into a table or 'flow chart' that enables you to clearly see the trend. Some wards will already use this method; if yours does not maybe you could introduce it.

Note-keeping

> . . . keep clear, accurate and legible records, reporting the relevant clinical findings, the decisions made, the information given to patients, and any drugs prescribed or other investigation or treatment . . . make records at the same time as the events you are recording or as soon as possible afterwards.[10]

The medical notes are the only way for each healthcare professional to find out the situation of each patient; so keep them contemporary, clear and accurate. Not only do medical notes serve as a communication tool for other professionals and to yourself, they are also there to protect you, and are a record that can be referred to during future claims or investigations. Think about every set of notes as potential evidence for a court case. Although it is a shame to practise defensive medicine, you will appreciate it if a patient sues three years down the line when you do not even remember their face, let alone your management of their condition. If notes are required as evidence, they will be photocopied. Therefore, always write medical notes in blue or, preferably, black pen. Never use green (the pharmacist's colour) or red (usually used for theatre notes) as, apart from being used by other professionals, these colours do not show up as well when copied.

> Abbreviations in medical records can lead to mistakes and misunderstandings.[13]

All entries in medical notes should be accompanied by a time and date. Do not add information to a past entry. If you do, put a date, time and signature next to this addition. Never cross out mistakes totally (e.g. by scribbling through it or using a correction fluid). Put a line through the incorrect word or sentence so the writing underneath is still legible.

Do not use acronyms in notes, this can lead to confusion and may potentially harm patients. Similarly, abbreviations should not be used, including the words 'left' and 'right', which are commonly written 'L' and 'R', respectively. If your handwriting is untidy, write in capitals. This goes for drug charts as well. Capital letters are often much clearer and their use reduces the chance of misunderstandings.

Specifically, write down what management is required and for when. Note down any medications or treatments that are stopped or started with an explanation for each decision. This will help in the future. Has the patient tried X before? Why did X not work? Why was X started? This information should also be included in discharge summaries for GPs.

Finish any entry in medical notes with your signature (and counter-signature if you are still a medical student), printed name, grade and bleep number (if appropriate).

Remember: if it is not in the notes then it did not happen.

Ill patients

During the day you may see someone whose condition is becoming unstable. Listen to the concerns of nurses and give the patient your full attention. Most of the jobs in a day could safely be left until later; your priority should be the sick patient. Remember, no one will criticise you if you have not written blood results in the notes, but they will do so if you ignored a sick patient. Every time you are called to see a patient, record your findings, actions and management plan in the notes.

Check the jobs book

Many wards have a doctor's jobs book, which detail the non-urgent jobs for that ward, for example re-writing drug charts. Try to check the job book regularly, especially if you have nothing much to do. You can often get ahead of yourself by completing these (often menial) tasks in a timely fashion. In addition, the doctor who is on call during the night will not thank you for leaving them lots of administrative jobs from the previous day!

Handover

At the end of the day, contact the junior doctor who is on call during the evening or night and 'handover' the patients you are most worried about. Inform the doctor of the patient's name, unit number, condition, management plan and any immediate concerns. Try to give a clear indication of how sick the patient is and how soon they need to be seen. Do not feel guilty for handing things over. It is better for the on-call doctor to receive this prior warning rather than being contacted in an emergency in the middle of the night for something they know nothing about.

> The transition from medical student to junior doctor is one of the most demanding phases of a medical career. The junior doctor years are associated with a variety of stressors, which can make doctors vulnerable to several important psychological and medical illnesses.[14]

Tips for maintaining your sanity during your time as a junior doctor

Prepare

Make the most of being a medical student. The best way to survive being a junior doctor is to get plenty of experience and exposure to the job while you are an undergraduate. Take time to not only shadow the consultants but also the junior staff.

Do not be hard on yourself

Every new doctor, at some point, feels like a fraud and wonders how they ever managed to graduate. Sometimes a lump appears in your throat, your bottom lip will wobble and you quickly seek sanctuary in a cupboard for a quick cry. Have comfort in the knowledge that every junior doctor has been through this. Take a break, go to the mess, have a coffee and moan to your peers about what a bad day you are having. When you are calm, go back to do what you are trained for, being a doctor!

Ask for help when you need it

In the first few days everything is new and you may feel out of your depth. Do not worry about asking for help. This is important for patient safety and the GMC states that doctors should recognise their own limitations and ask for help when required. Adopt puppy dog eyes, lose your arrogance and pride and look slightly lost; most people will be happy to assist.

Home time

An important part of the day that is often ignored by new doctors. Continually staying late after work is not sustainable and doing this will turn you into a quivering wreck. Remain an integrated member of society, maintain your hobbies and contact with the outside world and introduce a time limit on medical talk at home if you live with doctors.

USEFUL RESOURCES

Professional Medical

Graduated? First-shift butterflies? Professional Medical Education (PME) (www. freefees.co.uk) has designed a course targeted specifically at new doctors to help them get through their first few days and to give them a foundation for a brilliant career. The 'FY1 – Guide for the Uninitiated' course runs immediately prior to the beginning of the intake of new Foundation doctors, and covers:

➡ the team and your role within it
➡ common calls and how to confidently manage them
➡ emergencies – from asthma to diabetic ketoacidosis to a life-threatening bleed
➡ peri-operative management of the surgical patient
➡ how to impress your consultant
➡ research and audit – get involved!
➡ learn how to brush up your CV writing skills and discover how to perform at interview on the specialised PME courses – you'll knock 'em dead!

British Medical Association

The British Medical Association (BMA) runs fairs to assist your career development. The *British Medical Journal* (BMJ) Careers Fair (*see* www.bmjcareersfair.com and www.bma.org.uk/conferences) is an annual career fair, traditionally held in London in November. Since 2006 fairs are also held in Ireland, Wales, Scotland and the West Midlands. Free information, advice and support on your career are available. Workshops and seminars can be attended at an extra charge. Similar workshops are available at the BMA and BMJ Careers Skills Builder day. In 2006 these workshops were held in May. Workshops include CV skills, interview techniques and give advice specifically relating to filling out Foundation applications and how to move your career on. Reductions are given to BMA members.

Medical Protection Society Foundation programme resources

If you subscribe, for a small fee, to be a member of the Medical Protection Society (MPS) (www.mps.org.uk/foundationyears) in your Foundation years, you will be entitled to some useful benefits. In addition to medico-legal advice, support and representation, you will receive the journal, *Casebook*, on a quarterly basis, which contains information on risk management, case reports and news. You will also be eligible for a discount on some revision resources for your postgraduate exams and you will have access to an online clinical Foundation programme. The online clinical Foundation programme is provided by www.doctors.net.uk and consists of more than 40 interactive, educational modules that are related to your Foundation programme.

Medical Defence Union Foundation programme preparation

In July 2006, the Medical Defence Union (MDU) ran a one-day course in London on 'how to be a better house officer'. The fee for the course was reduced for MDU members. If you have concerns, queries or little confidence prior to starting your FY1 jobs, a course like this could be useful. In 2006 the course covered assessing and managing patients, emergencies, practical skills, filling in death certificates and drug charts and radiological interpretation. Look on the website (www.the-mdu. com/studentm) for up-to-date information and course content.

The Foundation Years journal

The Foundation Years is a bi-monthly journal, published by The Medicine Publishing Company, which is designed especially for Foundation doctors. The content of the journal covers the main competencies, both clinical and professional, that are required of junior doctors. A charge applies for the joint subscription of *The Foundation Years* and the *Medicine* journals. More information on charges, package details and sample articles can be found on the website (www.medicinejournal. co.uk).

BMJ Learning Foundation programme website

The *BMJ Learning* Foundation Programme website (www.bmjlearning.com/ foundation/index.htm) has been designed to assist your progress, learning and training throughout your Foundation years. It contains self-assessment forms to direct your experience, assist in reflective practice and help you present evidence of your competencies. You can complete forms online to monitor your progress and you can construct a personal development plan via the website. The website is easy to navigate and may really help you to organise your targets for the Foundation years.

'Am a House Officer Get Me Out of Here'

'Am a House Officer Get Me Out of Here' is a two-day course designed specifically for FY1 doctors (there is also one available for FY2 doctors). The course runs over a weekend and the fee (£200 in 2006) is reduced if you book both days. The first day of the course includes data interpretation (e.g. ECGs, blood tests/arterial blood gases and flow volume loops). The second day comprises a symptom-based approach to daily problems. The course incorporates evidence-based medicine and National Institute for Health and Clinical Excellence (NICE) guidelines. For more information and details on application visit the website (www.ceandt.co.uk/courses-houseofficer-course.asp).

Recommended books

There are many books for junior doctors. Indeed, many of the books you used throughout medical school will be helpful. Some more specific and widely used books are listed below. These books contain information about even the small, mundane jobs you may have to do as a junior doctor which you may not have asked about when you were a medical student. Do not forget, the defence organisations may provide you with some of these books free of charge if you sign up to be a member during your Foundation 1 year.

➥ Donald A, Stein M. *The Hands-on Guide for Junior Doctors*, 3rd ed. Oxford: Blackwell Publishing; 2006.

➥ Sanders S, Dawson J, Datta S, Eccles S. *Oxford Handbook for the Foundation Programme*. Oxford: Oxford University Press; 2005.

➥ Witham M, Jeetley P. *Crash Course House Officer's Guide*. Edinburgh: Mosby; 2004.

EDUCATION: IT NEVER ENDS

Do not make the mistake of thinking graduation is the end to your studying. When you are a postgraduate professional, education is known as 'continuing professional development' (CPD). You are required to learn and revise new and old information.

Nobody is exempt from CPD. The process is increasingly easy; for example, the *British Medical Journal* (BMJ) has developed the *BMJ Learning* website (www.bmjlearning.com), which contains interactive tutorials and personalised learning plans. You can construct your learning needs and undertake appropriate modules, record your progress and any notes you want to make. Similarly, the Doctors.net website (www.doctors.net.uk) has interactive tutorials for doctors covering a wide range of topics.

You may have the opportunity to attend specialty-specific conferences. If they are relevant to your work these can be invaluable as you gain the opportunity to hear the very latest research and speak to eminent professionals in your field

Journals encourage CPD by publishing new and, sometimes, groundbreaking research. Others even have CPD questions to test how well you have retained the information provided (e.g. those that accompany the journal *Medicine*, www.medicinecpd.co.uk).

WHAT MAY THE FUTURE HOLD?

There are many whisperings of what the future may hold, not just for doctors but for the NHS. Until they happen, speculations about changes are often inaccurate or misunderstood. Just make sure you keep abreast of potential changes and investigate anything that applies to you thoroughly. Some potential changes include the following.

➟ Revalidation of doctors by the General Medical Council. How and when (may be every five years) is unknown, but if this were to occur it would be crucial that you found out about it.

➟ Further changes to the Foundation programme application process. The junior doctor application process has changed substantially and annually since the early 1990s. Changes may be simple, including improved communication,[5] or more substantial, including major changes to the process itself, methods of application and scoring of applicants.[5] Communication of the application process has already changed as a timetable of application events is published on the application website well in advance of the application process opening.

➟ Increased number of doctors being in non-training posts. The prospect of this has already lowered the morale of many junior doctors. Make sure you are a good applicant by undertaking projects and activities that will boost your image on paper from a very early stage.

FURTHER READING

Alexander L. *Medicine Uncovered*. Richmond: Trotman; 2003.

Bolsin S. *100 or So Ways to Make your House Jobs/Internship Easier*, 1st ed. (Available from: www.juniordoctor.org productions.)

Cottrell E, Rebora C, Williams M. *The Medical Student Career Handbook*. Oxford: Radcliffe Publishing Ltd; 2006.

Donald A, Stein M, Muthu V. *The Hands-on Guide for House Officers*, 2nd ed. Oxford: Blackwell Science Ltd; 2002.

Foundation Programme Rough Guide (Available from: www.mmc.nhs.uk/pages/foundation/rough-guide www.labtestsonline.org [contains information on laboratory tests and conditions].)

Middleton J. *High-impact CVs: make your resume sensational*. Oxford: Infinite Ideas; 2005.

Modernising Medical Careers Working Group for Career Management. *Career Management: an approach for medical schools, deaneries, royal colleges and trusts*. London: Department of Health; 2005.

National Health Service Modernisation Agency, National Health Service National Patient Safety Agency, British Medical Association Junior Doctors Committee. *Safe Handover: safe patients. Guidance on clinical handover for clinicians and managers*. London: British Medical Association; 2004.

Witham M, Jeetley P. *Crash Course: house officer's guide*. Edinburgh: Mosby; 2004.

USEFUL WEBSITES

www.doctorjob.com/medicine/ (Doctor Job website)

www.maximizeyourmedicalcareer.com (Information on courses tailored to the most current job application processes.)

www.nes.scot.nhs.uk (Contains information on GP and specialist training schemes in Scotland)

Epilogue

Writing this book coincided with the end of my journey as a medical student. I have been through relationship break-ups, a marriage, joining the housing ladder, medical students from hell, tutors from heaven, new friendships, academic prizes, aggressive patients, personal illness, research, writing articles, money worries, two different part-time jobs and changing locations. This diversity will be familiar to you. It is only when you reach the end of your student life do you look back and realise just how much you have been through and you feel proud that you have come out the other end relatively unscathed.

I have had many highs and lows during medical school. These have helped me to be honest in the *Survival Guides*. The contributions of UK medical students have taught me that my experiences were not unique and I should not have felt alone. I hope that this book does the same for you and it helps you through your journey to being a doctor. Know you have company when the going gets tough.

You have already made the right steps. Reading this book will make you better informed of what lies ahead. I hope that your time as a medical student and as a doctor enriches your lives to the same extent as it has done mine. I feel grateful and honoured to have shared in the lives of so many patients and, through this book, medical students.

Best wishes for your future.

Resources

TALKING WITH PATIENTS AND COLLEAGUES

Professional Medical Education
Tel: 0800 043 2060
E-mail: courses@freefees.co.uk
Website: www.freefees.co.uk

HOW TO GET THE MOST FROM MEDICAL SCHOOL

Trauma conference for medical students
E-mail: enquires@traumamedicine.org
Website: www.traumamedicine.org

St Bart's and The Royal London Student Association Clubs
Union Building
Stepney Way
London E1 2AD

ELECTIVES

British Medical Association Services
Tel: 0845 010 1120
Website: www.bmas.co.uk

Institute for International Medical Education
750 Third Avenue
23rd Floor
New York
NY 10017
USA
E-mail: insitute@iime.org
Website: www.iime.org

WHEN THINGS GO WRONG

Anorexia Bulimia Care (ABC)
PO Box 173
Letchworth
Herts SG6 1XQ
Tel: 0146 242 3351
E-mail: anorexiabulimiacare@ntlworld.com
Website: www.anorexiabulimiacare.co.uk

BMA Counselling Service
Tel: 0845 920 0169 (local rates apply) open anytime, day or night, 365 days a year

BMA Doctors for Doctors Unit
Tel: 020 7383 6739

Doctors' SupportLine
38 Harwood Road
London SW6 4PH
(Generally open at the following times: Mon–Tue 6 pm to 11 pm; Wed–Fri 6 pm to
10 pm; Sun 10 am to 10 pm; Sat closed)
Tel: 0870 765 0001
Website: www.doctorssupport.org

Doctors' Support Network (DSN)
PO Box 360
Stevenage
Herts SG1 9AS
Tel: 0870 321 0642
Website: www.dsn.org.uk

Doctors' Support Network (DSN)
Wales and South-West
5 Borage Close
Pontprenneau
Cardiff CF23 8SJ
Tel: 0870 321 0642 or 0292 073 1025 (for administrative enquiries)

Eating Disorders Association
103 Prince of Wales Road
Norwich NR1 1DW
Tel: 0845 634 1414 (helpline) or 0870 770 3256 (for administrative enquiries)
E-mail: infor@edauk.com
Website: www.edauk.com

Mental Health Foundation
www.mentalhealth.org.uk

Mind
Mental health charity in England and Wales
Tel: 0845 766 0163
Website: www.mind.org.uk

Samaritans
Chris
PO Box 9090
Stirling FK8 2SA
Tel: 0845 790 9090; 185 060 9090 (Republic of Ireland)
Website: www.samaritans.org.uk

Sick Doctors Trust
Tel: 0870 444 5163
Website: www.sick-doctors-trust.co.uk

Support4Doctors
Website: www.support4doctors.org

LIFE AFTER MEDICAL SCHOOL

Professional Medical Education
Tel: 0800 043 2060
E-mail: courses@freefees.co.uk
Website: www.freefees.co.uk

References

Note to Chapter 1: Introduction

1 Royal College of Physicians. *Doctors in Society: medical professionalism in a changing world*. Report of a working party of the Royal College of Physicians of London. London: Royal College of Physicians; 2005.

Notes to Chapter 2: Clinical years

1 Powell M. *The Little Book of Crap Advice*. London: Michael O'Mara Books; 2001.

2 Barrie M. *The Surgeon's Rhyme: a memoir*. Lewes: The Book Guild; 2004.

3 Council of Heads of Medical Schools and British Medical Association Medical Students Committee. Medical Student Charter, 2005. (Available at: www.bma. org.uk/ap.nsf/Content/MedSchCharter)

4 The Housing (Management of Houses in Multiple Occupations) Regulations. London: HMSO; 1990.

5 Clarke R. Ethical Grid, 2004. (Available at: www.askdoctorclarke.com)

6 Beasley R, Robinson G, Aldington S. From medical student to junior doctor: accepting the responsibility of informed consent. *StudentBMJ*. 2006; **14**: 9–6.

7 General Medical Council. *Seeking Patients' Consent: the ethical considerations*. London: General Medical Council; 1998.

8 Holden J. *Hot Topic: students and consent*. London: Medical Defence Union; 2006.

9 General Medical Council. *Confidentiality: protecting and providing information*. London: General Medical Council; 2004.

10 General Medical Council. *Tomorrow's Doctors: recommendations on undergraduate medical education*. London: General Medical Council; 2003.

11 Lill MM, Wilkinson TJ. Judging a book by its cover: descriptive survey of patients' preferences for doctors' appearance and mode of address. *BMJ*. 2005; **331**: 1524–7.

12 Rehman SU, Nietert PJ, Cope DW, Kilpatrick AO. What to wear today? Effect of doctors' attire on the trust and confidence of patients. *Am J Med*. 2005; **118**: 1279–86.

Notes to Chapter 3: Talking with patients and colleagues

1 Rubin P. *Core Education Outcomes: GMC Education Committee position statement.* London: General Medical Council; 2006.

2 Tyler KM. Peer-level multiple source feedback for fitness to practice. *Med Educ.* 2006; **40**: 482–3.

3 National Health Service Modernisation Agency, National Health Service National Patient Safety Agency, British Medical Association Junior Doctors Committee. *Safe Handover: safe patients. Guidance on clinical handover for clinicians and managers.* London: British Medical Association; 2005.

4 Laidlaw TS, Kaufman DM, MacLeod H, Zanten SV, Simpson D, Wrixon W. Relationship of resident characteristics, attitudes, prior training and clinical knowledge to communication skills performance. *Med Educ.* 2006; **40**: 18–25.

5 General Medical Council. *Tomorrow's Doctors: recommendations on undergraduate medical education.* London: General Medical Council; 2003. (Available from: www.gmc-uk.org)

6 Haynes K, McTigue A. Just what the doctor ordered. *Casebook.* 2006; **14**: 8–10.

7 Baile WF, Buckman R, Lenzi R, Glober G, Beale EA, Kudelka AP. SPIKES. A six step protocol for delivering bad news: application to the patient with cancer. *Oncologist.* 2000; **5**: 302–11.

8 Langewitz W, Denz M, Keller A, Kiss A, Rüttimann S, Wössmer B. Spontaneous talking time at start of consultation in outpatient clinic: cohort study. *BMJ.* 2002; **325**: 682–3.

Notes to Chapter 4: History-taking

1 Porter R. *Blood and Guts: a short history of medicine.* London: Allen Lane; 2002.

2 Hampton J. Relative contribution of history taking, physical examination and the laboratory to the diagnosis and management of medical outpatients. *BMJ.* 1975; **2**: 486.

3 General Medical Council. *Tomorrow's Doctors: recommendations on undergraduate medical education.* London: General Medical Council; 2003.

4 http://en.wikipedia.org/wiki/William_Osler

Notes to Chapter 5: Examination of patients

1 Rubin P. *Core Education Outcomes: GMC Education Committee position statement.* London: General Medical Council; 2006.

2 General Medical Council. *Tomorrow's Doctors: recommendations on undergraduate medical education.* London: General Medical Council; 2003.

3 General Medical Council. *Intimate Examinations.* London: General Medical Council; 2001.

4 Kavanagh S, Anthony S. Close encounters of the risky kind. *MPS Casebook.* 2004; **12**: 13–14.

5 Stern V. Gynaecological examinations post-Ledward? a private matter. *Lancet.* 2001; **358**: 1896–8.

6 Barrie M. *The Surgeon's Rhyme: a memoir.* Lewes: The Book Guild; 2004.

Note to Chapter 6: Presenting patients

1 General Medical Council. *Tomorrow's Doctors: recommendations on undergraduate medical education.* London: General Medical Council; 2003.

Notes to Chapter 7: Ward life and rounds

1 General Medical Council. *Tomorrow's Doctors: recommendations on undergraduate medical education.* London: General Medical Council; 2003.

2 Sithamparanthan M. 'enthusiastic, hard-working, a good team player . . .' Is teamwork working in the NHS? *GMC Today.* 2005; **5**: 6–7.

3 Gleeson FV. The chest radiograph in heart disease. *Medicine.* 2006; **34**: 136–41.

Note to Chapter 10: Community placements

1 General Medical Council. *Tomorrow's Doctors: recommendations on undergraduate medical education.* London: General Medical Council; 2003.

Note to Chapter 11: How to get the most from medical school

1 Council of Heads of Medical Schools and British Medical Association Medical Students Committee. Medical Student Charter, 2005. (Available at: www.bma. org.uk/ap.nsf/Content/MedSchCharter)

Notes to Chapter 12: Electives

1 Council of Heads of Medical Schools and British Medical Association Medical Students Committee. Medical Student Charter, 2005. (Available at: www.bma. org.uk/ap.nsf/Content/MedSchCharter)

2 Wilson M. *The Medic's Guide to Work and Electives around the World,* 2nd ed. Oxford: Arnold Publishers; 2004.

3 www.fco.gov.uk/travel

4 British Medical Association. *Medicine in the 21st Century: standards for the delivery of undergraduate medical education.* London: BMA; 2005.

5 Chaudry E, Aslam A. The crown jewel of medical school. *StudentBMJ.* 2006; **14**: 286–7.

6 British Medical Association, Royal Pharmaceutical Society of Great Britain. *British National Formulary,* 51st ed. London: BMJ Publishing Group Ltd and RPS Publishing; 2006.

7 Madge S, Matthews P, Singh S. *HIV in Primary Care: an essential guide to HIV for GPs, practice nurses and other members of the primary healthcare team.* London: Medical Foundation for AIDS and Sexual Health; 2004. www.medfash.org. uk/publications/documents/HIV_in_Primary_Care.pdf

8 www.qub.ac.uk/cm/mednews/y4/elective-0607.htm

Notes to Chapter 13: When things go wrong

 1 Powell M. *The Little Book of Crap Advice*. London: Michael O'Mara Books; 2001.
 2 Advisory, Conciliation and Arbitration Service. *Religion or Belief and the Workspace: putting the employment equality (religion or belief) regulations 2003 into practice*. London: ACAS; 2004.
 3 Wood D. Bullying and harassment in medical schools. *BMJ*. 2006; **333**: 664–5.
 4 Health Policy and Economic Research Unit. *Medical Students' Welfare Survey: report*. London: British Medical Association; 2006.
 5 Paice E, Aitken M, Houghton A, Firth-Cozens J. Bullying among doctors in training: cross sectional questionnaire survey. *BMJ*. 2005; **329**: 658–9.
 6 McManus IC, Richards P, Winder BC, Sproston KA. Clinical experience, performance in final examinations, and learning style in medical students: prospective study. *BMJ*. 1998; **316**: 345–50.
 7 General Medical Council. *Good Medical Practice*. London: General Medical Council; 2006. (Available from: www.gmc-uk.org/med-ed/default.htm)
 8 Hebert K. Cover up. *StudentBMJ*. 2005; **13**: 298–9.
 9 British Medical Association Central Consultants and Specialists Committee. *Tackling Racism in Medical Careers: the role of consultants – policy paper*. London: British Medical Association; 2005.
10 Smith GB, Poplett N. Knowledge of aspects of acute care in trainee doctors. *Postgrad Med J*. 2002; **78**: 335–8.
11 Resuscitation Council (UK). *Advanced Life Support*. London: Resuscitation Council (UK); 2006.
12 www.qub.ac.uk/cm/mednews/y4/elective-0607.htm
13 Bell DM. Occupational risk of HIV virus infection in health care workers: an overview. *Am J Med*. 1997; **102**: 9–15.
14 Handerson DK. Postexposure prophylaxis for occupational exposures to hepatitis B, hepatitis C and HIV virus. *Surg Clin North Am*. 1995; **75**: 1175–87.
15 Centers for Disease Control and Prevention. Recommendation for prevention and control of HCV infection and HCV related chronic disease. *MMWR Morb Mortal Wkly Rep*. 1998; **47**: 1.
16 General Medical Council. *Serious Communicable Diseases*. London: General Medical Council; 1997.

Notes to Chapter 14: Difficult individuals

 1 Butler CC, Evans M, The Welsh Philosophy and General Practice Discussion Group. The 'heartsink' patient revisited. *Br J Gen Prac*. 1999; **49**: 230–3.
 2 Robinson G, Beasley R, Aldington S. From medical student to junior doctor: the 'difficult patient'. *StudentBMJ*. 2006; **14**: 278–9.

Notes to Chapter 15: *Life after medical school*

1 www.mmc.nhs.uk/download_files/Curriculum-for-the-foundation-years-in-postgraduate-education-and-training.pdf

2 www.mmc.nhs.uk/download/MMC%20Past-Future7.pdf

3 www.mmc.nhs.uk/pages/foundation/foundation-learning-portfolio

4 Powell M. *The Little Book of Crap Advice*. London: Michael O'Mara Books; 2001.

5 British Medical Association Medical Students Committee. *Medical Students' Annual Report*. London: British Medical Association; 2006.

6 Kmietowicz Z. Doctors defend online system for allocating junior doctor posts. *StudentBMJ*. 2006; **14**: 182.

7 Palmer R, Howes J. Internet recruitment of foundation year 1 programmes. *BMJ Career Focus*. 2005; **331**: 263–4.

8 Pritchard L. First-time fiasco for 'fairer' web job hunt. *Student BMA News*. 2006; 1. (Available from: www.bma.org.uk/ap.nsf/Content?Hubstudentbmanews)

9 British Medical Association. *Medical Students: widening participation in medical schools*. London: British Medical Association; 2004. (Available at: www.bma.org.uk/ap.nsf/Content/Medstudparticipation)

10 General Medical Council. *Good Medical Practice*. London: General Medical Council; 2006. (Available from: www.gmc-uk.org/med-ed/default.htm)

11 Council of Heads of Medical Schools and British Medical Association Medical Students Committee. Medical Student Charter, 2005. (Available from: www.bma.org.uk/ap.nsf/Content/MedSchCharter)

12 Sithamparanathan M. 'enthusiastic, hard-working, a good team player . . .' Is teamwork working in the NHS. *GMC Today*. 2005; **5**: 6–7.

13 Stewart H. *Abbreviations Should be Avoided in Medical Records*. London: Medical Defence Union; 2006.

14 Robinson G, Bernau S, Aldington S, Beasley R. From medical student to junior doctor: maintaining good health during the 'baptism of fire'. *StudentBMJ*. 2006; **14**: 138–9.

Index